THE FIRST COMPLETE BOOK ON VIBRATION
PLATE EXERCISE PROGRAMS
STEP BY STEP
EASY TO FOLLOW

MOHSEN KAZEMI

VIBRATION PLATE EXERCISES

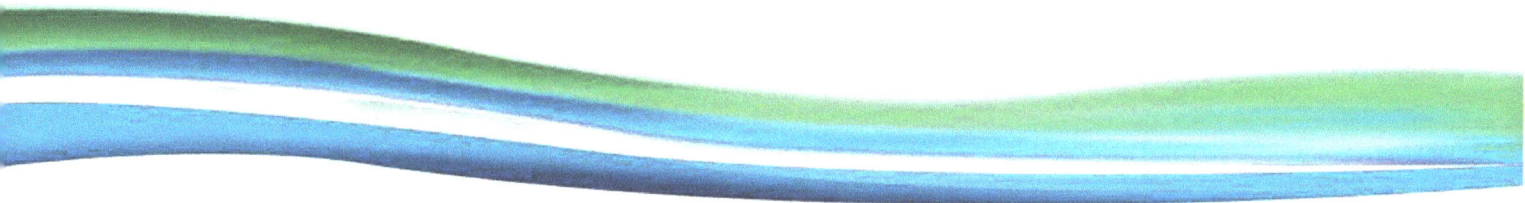

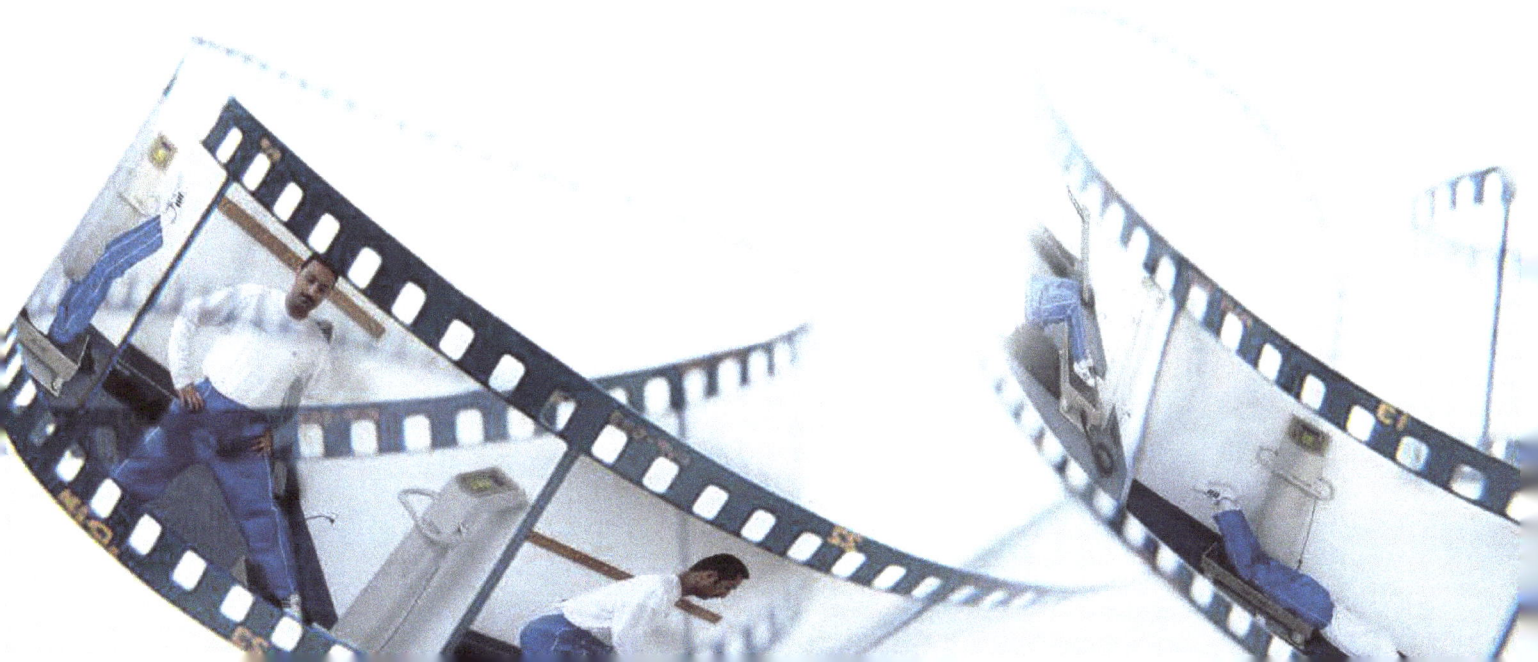

Printed in Ontario, Canada

DISCLAIMER: This book is designed for the purpose of education the reader in regards to the subject matter covered. The information is not intended for medical diagnosis, nor should it be relied upon to recommend a treatment protocol for an individual. The author is not responsible in any manner, whatsoever, for any injury or loss that may result following the information contained within this book. The exercises described may be too strenuous or dangerous for some people and the reader should consult their physician or other qualified health care practitioner before engaging in a new exercise regime. If you are suffering from Deep Vein Thrombosis (DVT), infection, inflammation, dizziness, cancer or cardiovascular disease, consult your family physician or other qualified health care professionals prior to engaging in the exercises outlined in this book. Never ignore medical advice or delay in seeking it because of something contained in this book.

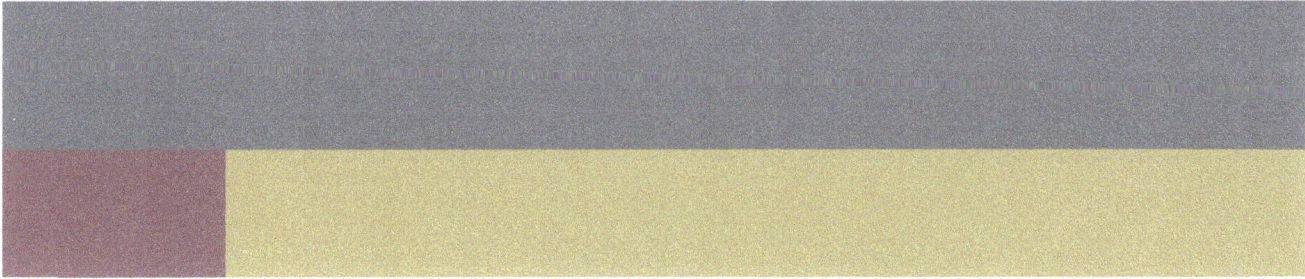

DEDICATION

This book is dedicated to my beloved wife, Insook for her unconditional love, support, and unfailing encouragement.

ABOUT THE AUTHOR

Dr. Mohsen Kazemi, R.N., D.C., D.Ac, F.C.C.S.S.(C), D.A.C.R.B.,F.C.C.R.S.(C)

Dr. Mohsen Kazemi is a Professor of Clinical Education and the coordinator of the Sports Sciences Residency program at the Canadian Memorial Chiropractic College (CMCC). He is a Fellow of the Royal College of Chiropractic Sports Sciences (Canada) and a Fellow of the College of Chiropractic and Physical and Occupational Rehabilitation (Canada). With 30 years of experience in acupuncture, he has made significant contributions to both the academic and clinical fields.

Dr. Kazemi successfully defended his PhD thesis, titled "What Makes Sparing Taekwondo Athletes Successful," at South Wales University. He has published numerous articles in peer-reviewed journals and presented research on Taekwondo and chiropractic internationally. Dr. Kazemi is also an assistant editor for the Journal of the Canadian Chiropractic Association.

As an inventor, Dr. Kazemi created the VMTX Vibromax Therapeutics® soft tissue technique, the Kazemizer (a portable exercise device designed to prevent lactic acid buildup), the Kazemizer Shark® (an instrument-assisted soft tissue therapy mobilization tool), and the Leukomizer® Taping Technique.nted his research in Taekwondo, chiropractic, sports injuries and rehabilitation around the world.

Dr. Kazemi has served in numerous prestigious roles, including as the Alternate Chiropractor for the Core Canadian Health Care Team at the 2002 Winter Olympics in Salt Lake City, the 2002 Commonwealth Games in Manchester, the 2007 Pan American Games in Rio, and the 2008 Olympic Games in Beijing. He was also part of the Core Canadian Medical Team at the 2003 Pan American Games in Santo Domingo and served as the Chiropractor for the Canadian Taekwondo team at the 2008 Beijing and 2016 Rio Olympics. Additionally, Dr. Kazemi was the appointed Chiropractor for Mount Cypress at the 2010 Winter Olympics, the only Canadian Chiropractor at the first Youth Olympic Games in Singapore (2010), and the Chiropractor at the 2011 and 2015 Pan Am Games.

Since 2003, he has held the position of Medical Chair for the Ontario Taekwondo Association, was the Taekwondo Canada Medical Chair from 2009–2010, and served as the High-Performance IST (Integrated Support Team) Coordinator from 2015–2016. Dr. Kazemi has been the traveling team doctor and chiropractor for the Canadian Taekwondo National Team since 1998.

A Grand Master with an 8th-degree black belt in Taekwondo, Dr. Kazemi has been a Canadian Poomsae Taekwondo Champion for several years. He was also the Champion at the 2008 World Taekwondo Hanmadang and the 2017 Commonwealth Poomsae Championships. Additionally, he earned a silver medal at the 2008 Commonwealth Taekwondo Championships, the 2019 World Cup Poomsae, and the 2022 Pan Am Taekwondo Championships, as well as multiple bronze medals in the Pan Am Taekwondo Championships in 2012, 2014, 2016, 2018, 2020, and 2024.

CONTENTS

CHAPTER 1 .... 01 - 02
What is Whole Body Vibration(WBV)

CHAPTER 2 .... 03 - 08
Lower Body Exercises

CHAPTER 3 .... 09 - 14
Core Exercises

CHAPTER 4 .... 15 - 20
Upper Body Exercises

CHAPTER 5 .... 21 - 32
Beginners Programs

CHAPTER 6 .... 33 - 42
Bone Density Enhancement Programs

CHAPTER 7 .... 43 - 56
Full Body Programs

CHAPTER 8 .... 57 - 88
Sports Specific Programs

CHAPTER 9 .... 89 - 96
High Intensity Booth Camp Programs

CHAPTER 10 .... 97 - 106
Program Summary Tables

Frequently Asked Questions 107

References .... 108 - 112

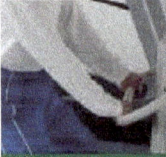

The Whole Body Vibration exercise programs are based on 30 years of research. Whole Body Vibration (WBV) was initially used in Europe in the late 1800's for exercise and therapeutic purposes. WBV has been used to treat bone and lean muscle mass loss in astronomers who spend considerable time in space. The WBV trainer is an oscillating platform with a frequency of 5 to 50 Hz. The WBV trainer induces vibration that transmits through muscles, bones and soft tissues. Each muscle in order to do its job of holding specific postures has to overcome the vibration first and then hold the position. Research shows to do this 95% of the muscle fibers have to fire. In addition, since the vibration transmits through the whole body there is no escape for all other muscles, bones and soft tissues of the body from the effect of vibration. Therefore, as a natural response they are all activated. This activation counts for overall increased metabolism and increase overall strength, power, endurance, decrease body fat, increase bone density, Growth Hormones (fountain of youth, elixir of life), testosterone (increase energy and reproduction), Serotonin and Dopamine (Happy Hormones), blood circulation (increase healing and metabolism), lymphatic drainage (removal of toxins and rejuvenating tissues) and neuromuscular enhancement (increase strength and power). This overall activation of all tissues counts for the fact that 10 minutes of exercises on WBV trainer is equal to 30-40 minutes of weight training. This makes WBV Exercise programs ideal for busy people who desire to keep active but do not have enough time.

WBV has been also used in athletic population extensively starting in Russia, Europe and now here in North America. Research indicates the same results have observed in Athletes as well as lay person. Competitive Athletes will gain the edge that they need to win in strength, power, endurance and overall performance participating in the WBV programs demonstrated in this book.

Falls are one of the most common causes of injury and death in elderly. Falls in elderly are usually as a result of decrease strength, balance and bone density. WBV program with its soft nature exercise, enhancing balance, hormones and bone density, is the perfect exercise for elderly who desire to increase their strength, balance, bone density and overall wellness. WBV is the only exercise shown recently to increase bone density in post-menopausal women 60-70 years old.

Specific WBV programs in this book are designed to help you achieve your goals, from increasing your bone density, losing weight, strengthening your core to specifically focusing and strengthening your upper or lower limbs.

Features : WBV programs

Muscles

- Increasing muscular strength
- Enhancing muscle flexibility
- Improving muscle elasticity
- Expediting recovery of muscle fatigue
- Relieving muscle pain

Joint, tendons, connective tissue

- Increasing muscle flexibility
- Decreasing adhesions

Blood Vessels

- Improving blood circulation
- Enhancing metabolism
- Reducing edema with muscle pump increase

1

Hormones

- Increasing growth hormones also known as youth hormones
- Increasing productivity of Testosterone hormones
- Reducing newly forming cortisol hormones also known as inflammatory hormones
- Increasing serotonin hormones and neurotophine so called happy hormones

Nervous System

- Improving sensitivity of nervous system

Skin

- Accelerating drainage to lymph and vessels with increased blood circulation
- Reducing cellulite
- Improving skin quality with increased muscle strength and collagen

Bone

- Preventing and healing osteoporosis

Fat

- Burning fat to reduce body fat
- Stimulating abdominal muscles and helping metabolism to reduce fat in abs area

BASIC PRINCIPLES

Whole Body Vibration (WBV) exercises are based on holding a specific position on the vibrating plate for a specific duration of time. Each position described in this book is designed to specifically target certain muscles. However, other parts (bone, ligaments and fascia) and muscles of the body are not exempted from getting stimulated by vibration and will be stimulated in lesser degrees.

In general, one would start with easier positions and work towards the harder and more challenging ones. The progression of holding each position would be from a short 10 seconds and working towards holding to maximum duration. When maximum hold time has been obtained, one can decrease the rest time between each exercise to increase the intensity of the programs. In addition, to focus and further strengthen an area you can repeat the specific exercise for this area three to four times with 30 to 60 seconds rest between each repetition. To further intensify the exercises you can hold hand held weights and assume the position, and or do each exercise in repetitive motion.

In summary:

- Hold specific position for specific muscles.
- Start from easy position and work towards more challenging ones.
- Start with holding a position for short time and work towards holding the position for full duration as recommended for each program.
- To further intensify each program once you reached the maximum hold time and felt comfortable, you can decrease the rest time between each exercise.

CHAPTER 2

LOWER BODY EXERCISES

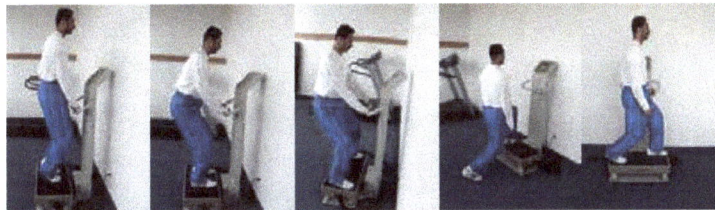

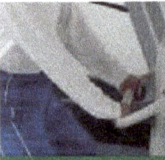

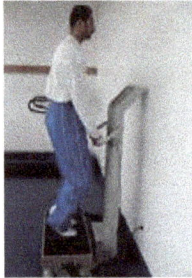

CALVES

Targets: Calves (gastroc, soleus, and tibialis posterior), gluteus maximus (glut max), quadriceps, hamstrings and back.

- Stand on your toes.
- For more balance you can hold on to the device handle bar.
- To improve your balance stand without holding to the handle.
- To train the larger calf muscles (gastorcs) straighten your knee.
- To train the deeper muscles of your calf bend your knees.
- To make this exercise harder, stand on one leg.

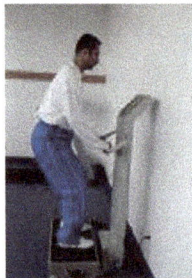

SQUAT

Targets: Quadriceps, glut max, calves and back.

- Stand with your hips and knees bent about 30 degrees and keep your back straight.
- For stability hold on to the handle bar.
- To train your balance, try to stand without holding on to the handle bar. (harder)
- To make this exercise more challenging stand on one leg.

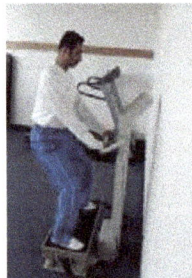

DEEP SQUAT

Targets: Quadriceps, glut max, calves and back.

- Stand with your knees and hips bent at 50 to 60 degrees and as you get use to it you can go as low as 90 degree.
- Keep your back straight.
- For stability hold on to the handle bar.
- To train your balance, try to stand without holding on to the handle bar. (harder)
- To make this exercise more challenging stand on one leg.

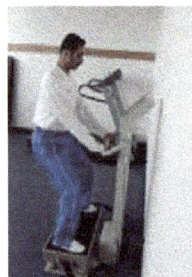

WIDE STANCE SQUAT

Targets: Quadriceps, glut max, calves and back.

- Stand with your feet to the edge of the plate with your knees and hips bent to 50-60 degrees.
- Keep your back straight.
- For stability hold on to the handle bar.
- To train your balance, try to stand without holding on to the handle bar.

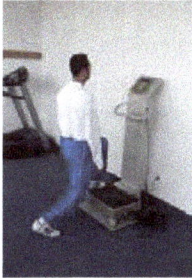

LUNGE

Targets: Hamstrings, quadriceps, hip flexors, glut max and med.

- Stand toward the trainer and one foot on the plate and the front knee bent to 90 degree.
- Your back knee can be slightly bent.
- To increase intensity of the exercise, bend the back knee further.
- Keep your back straight.

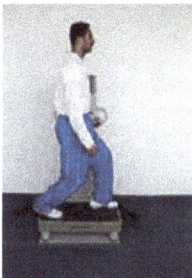

SIDE LUNGE

Targets: Hamstrings, quadriceps, glut max, hip flexors, calves & anterior shin.

- Stand side way on the plate as wide as your plate allows you.
- To increase the intensity, try to pinch the plate with your feet.
- For stability hold on to the handle bar.
- To train your balance, try to stand without holding on to the handle bar.

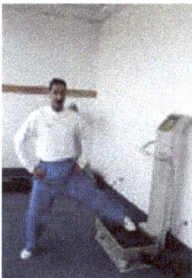

ADDUCTOR STRETCH

Targets: Hip adductors, hamstring & calf.

- Stand side way with one foot on the plate with the leg straight.
- Feel the stretch inside of your thigh.
- You can increase the stretch with bending the knee of the foot on the floor.

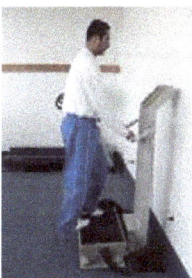

CALF STRETCH

Targets: Calves.

- Stand with your toes on the edge of the plate and the heel of the calf to stretch off the edge.
- To stretch the large calf muscles (gastrocs) keep the back knee straight.
- To stretch the deeper calf muscle (soleus), bend the back knee.

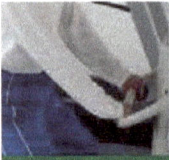

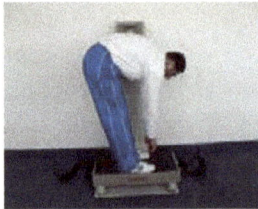

HAMSTRING STRETCH

Targets: Hamstrings, calves and back.

- Stand side ways of the plate.
- Bend forward and keep your knees straight.

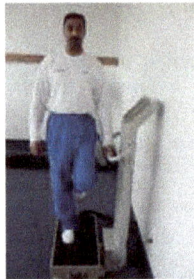

ONE LEGGED STANCE

Targets: Glut medius (med), minimus (min), and maximus (max), back and core muscles.

- Stand on the plate side ways on one leg.
- For stability hold on to the handle bar.
- To train your balance, try to stand without holding on to the handle bar.

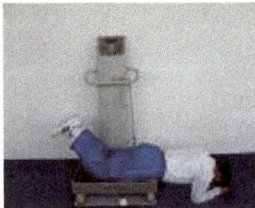

QUADRICEPS MASSAGE

Targets: Glut medius (med), minimus (min), and maximus (max), back and core muscles.

- To massage your thighs (quadriceps), lie on the plate face down with your thighs over the plate.
- Bend your knees slightly.

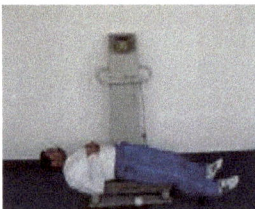

HAMSTRINGS MASSAGE

Targets: Glut medius (med), minimus (min), and maximus (max), back and core muscles.

- To massage your hamstrings, lie on your back with your hamstrings (back of your thighs) in contact with the plate.

2

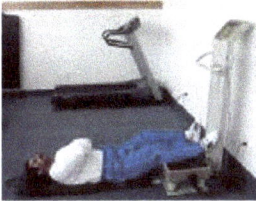

CALVES MASSAGE

Targets: Hamstrings, quadriceps, glut max, hip flexors, calves & anterior shin.

- To massage your calves, lie down on the floor with your calves on the plate.

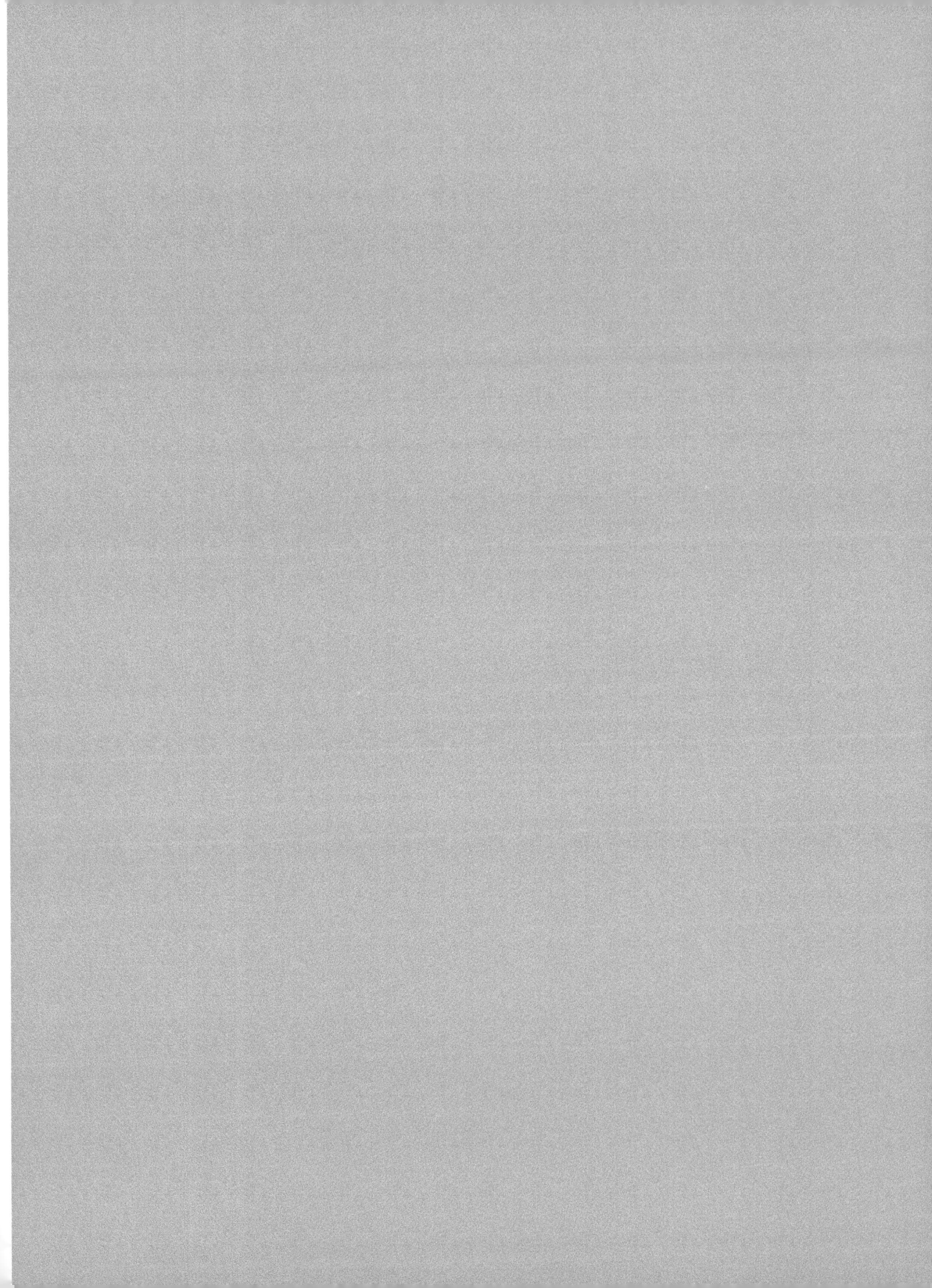

CHAPTER 3

CORE EXERCISES

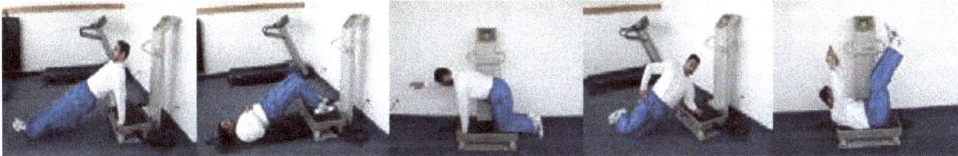

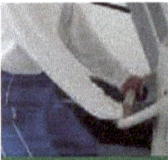

CHAPTER 3

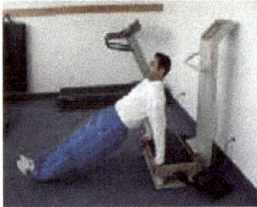

FRONT BRIDGE

Targets: Shoulders, triceps, abdominals, deep abdominals, back & hamstrings.

- Support yourself with your hands at the edge of the plate, facing up.
- Keep your body in one line and avoid bending at your waist.
- Keep your elbows straight

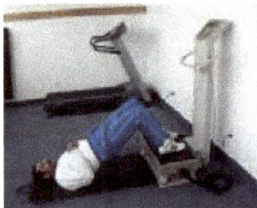

BACK BRIDGE

Targets: Abdominals, back muscles, gluts, hamstrings & calves.

- Lie down on the floor facing up.
- Put your feet on the plate and lift your pelvis off the floor.
- Keep your back and thighs in one line.

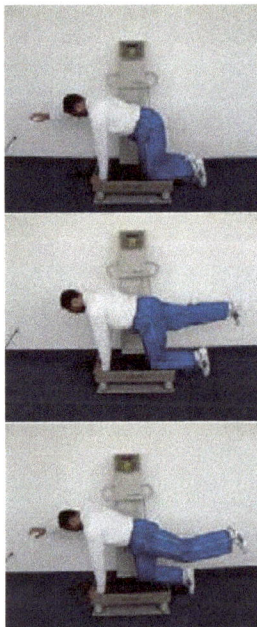

BRID DOG OR CROSS CRAWL

Targets: Back muscles and core low back and neck, glut max, hamstrings, shoulder stabilizing muscles, and balance.
Bird Dog or Cross Crawl exercises shown in the pictures can start with beginners lifting one arm and then one leg to more advance lifting opposite arm and leg.

- Put a mat or towel on the plate.
- Go on your fours, i.e. on your knees and hands over the plate.
- Keep your back and neck straight and do not look up.
- Lift one arm parallel to your body.
- Do not lift your arm above your head.
- Put your hand down and then lift one leg.
- Repeat the two above steps for other arm and leg and hold each position based on the program you are following.

Move on to do this position after you are comfortable with the beginners version.

- Go on your fours on the plate.
- Keep your back and neck in a straight line.
- Tuck your chin in order to train your deep neck flexors at the same time.
- Lift opposite arm and leg at the same time and hold according to your program.

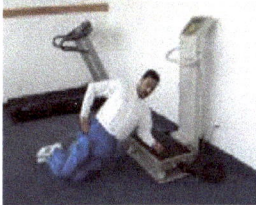

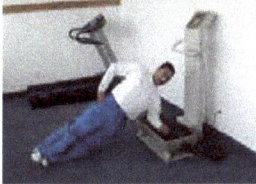

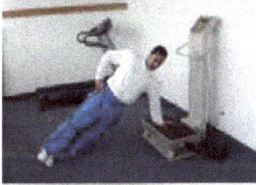

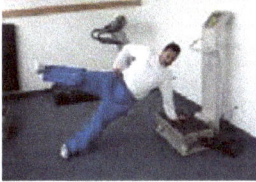

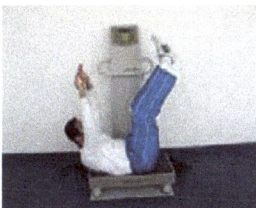

LATERAL RAISES

Targets: Deep lateral back muscles (quadratus lomborum), deep abdominals (internal obliquues and transversus abdominus), glut med and min, Iliotibial band (ITB), shoulder, arm & neck.

Lateral raises exercises can be progressed from simple to complex and more challenging as shown in the pictures sequentially. It is advisable to master each level before moving on to the next level.

- Assume side way position with your elbow on the plate.
- You can put a towel or a mat over the plate to decrease pressure over your elbow.
- For the beginners bend your knees and keep your body straight in one line as shown in the first picture.
- For the next level straighten your legs so that your contacts are your elbow and the side of your foot.
- For level three assume the side position with your hand on the plate keeping your arm straight.
- Keep your body in one line.
- For this ultimate side raise position, assume sideways position with your hand on the plate.
- Keep your arm straight.
- Keep your body in one line.
- Lift your leg toward the ceiling and hold.

DEAD BUG

Targets: Abdominals, deep abdominals, hip flexors, neck deep flexors, shoulders and back.

- Lie on your back on the plate.
- Lift your arms and legs straight.
- Tuck your chin and lift your head.

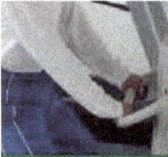

BACK EXTENSION

Targets: Back, scapular/shoulder stabilizing, neck extensors & glut max.

- Lie on your stomach on the plate.
- Put your hands behind your head.
- Lift your head, shoulders and legs off the plate and hold.
- To make this exercise more intense and challenging extend your arms in front of you in the same line of your body in SUPERMAN position.

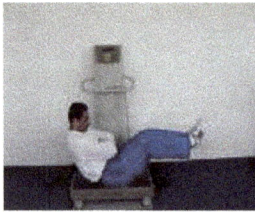

BASIC ABS

Targets: Abdominals, hip flexors & quadriceps.

- Lie on your back on the plate.
- Tuck your chin.
- Lift up your legs and back about 30 degrees off the plate and hold.
- Easier way would be to only lift your back or your legs.

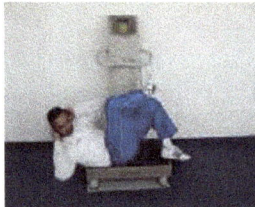

DIAGONAL ABS

Targets: External and internal oblique abdominals.

- Lie on your back on the plate.
- Put your hands behind your head and cross one leg over your knee.
- Twist and touch opposite elbow to opposite knee and hold.

Another modification of this exercise is:

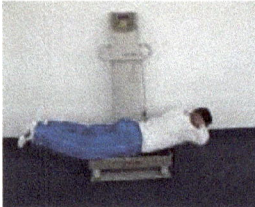

- Lie on your side on the plate.
- Lift your shoulder or your legs off the plate and hold.
- For more intensity lift your shoulders and legs off the floor together and hold.

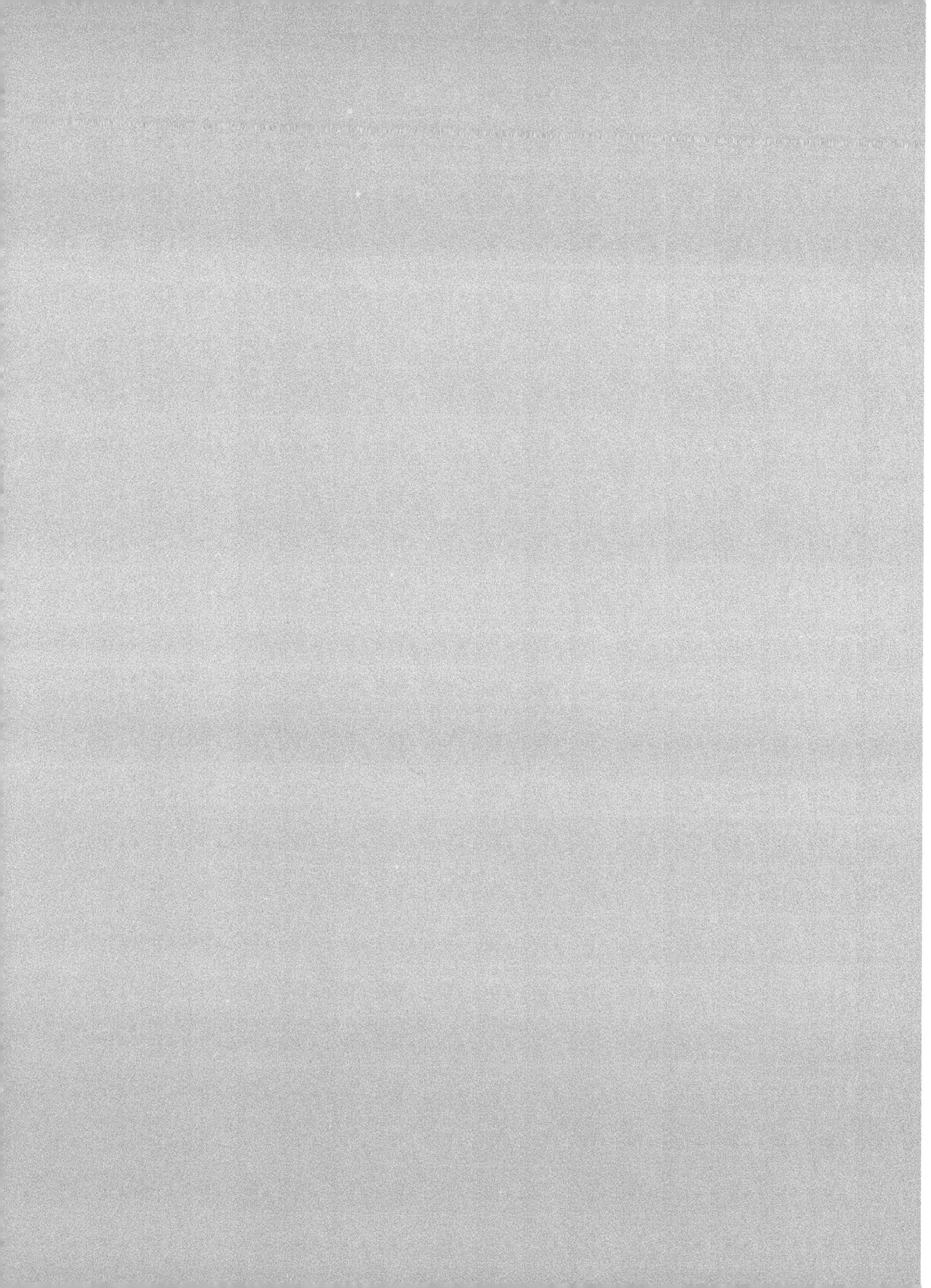

CHAPTER 4

UPPER BODY EXERCISES

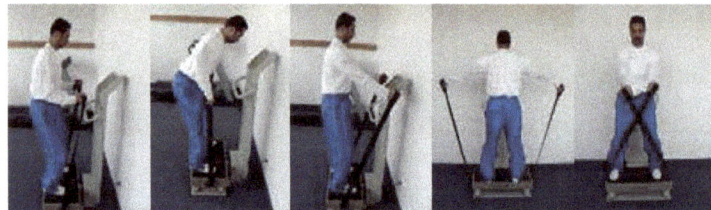

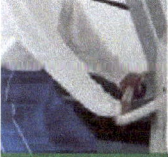

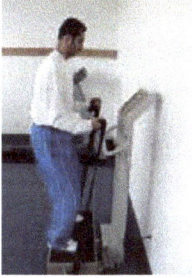

BICEPS CURLS

Targets: Biceps, anterior shoulder (deltoid), wrist flexors, quadriceps & gluts.

- Stand on the plate.
- Hold on the straps, which are attached to the side of the plate with your palms toward the ceiling.
- Bend your elbows to 90 degrees and pull on the straps upward.

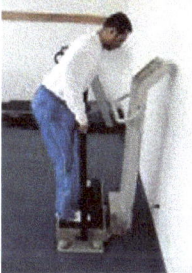

LATS

Targets: Lats (latisimus dorsi), triceps, posterior shoulder, quadriceps & gluts.

- Stand on the plate with your feet wide apart.
- Hold on to the straps palm down.
- Pull on the straps backward and up.

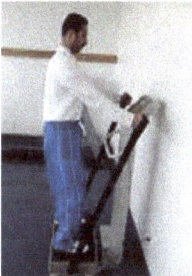

ANTERIOR DELT

Targets: Shoulder (Anterior deltoid), biceps, brachioradialis & trapezius.

- Stand on the plate and hold on to the straps palms facing one another.
- Keep your elbow straight and pull the straps towards the ceiling.

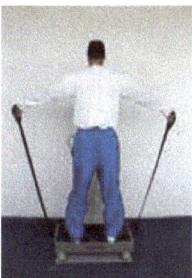

LATERAL DELT

Targets: Lateral shoulder (lateral deltoid), triceps, wrist extensors & trapezius.

- Stand on the plate with your feet shoulder width apart.
- Hold on to the straps with your thumbs facing the floor and pull on them upward parallel to your body.

4

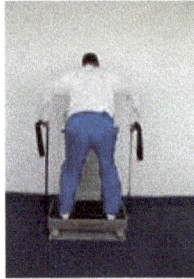

POSTERIOR DELT

Targets: Posterior shoulders (posterior deltoid), triceps, scapular stabilizers (rhomboids, mid and lower trapezius), quadriceps & gluts.

- Stand on the plate with your feet shoulder width apart.
- Bend your knees about 50 degrees and bend forward about 40 degrees.
- Hold on to the straps with your elbows bent at 90 degrees.
- Pull on the straps backwards and try to squeeze your shoulder blades together at the same time.

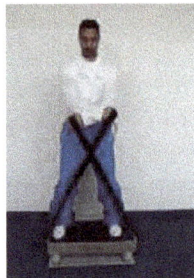

PEC CROSS

Targets: Chest (pectoralis), biceps, wrist flexors, & anterior shoulder (anterior deltoid).

- Stand on the plate with your feet wide apart.
- Grab the straps, bend your elbows and cross your arms.
- Pull on the straps towards your opposite shoulders.

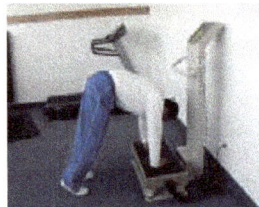

SHOULDER PRESS

Targets: Shoulders (anterior and lateral deltoids), trapezius, wrist flexors and extensors, & scapular stabilizers.

- Stand on the floor and bend over with your hands on the plate.
- Keep your hands shoulder width apart.
- Keep your elbows straight.
- To increase the intensity, shift your weight onto your arms by going on your toes.

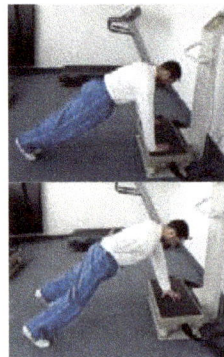

PUSH UP

Targets: Chest (pectoralis), shoulders (anterior, lateral and posterior deltoid), biceps, triceps, serratus anterior, rhomboids, back and abdominal.

- Put your hands on the plate shoulder width apart.
- Keep your feet together on the floor.
- Keep your body straight in one line.
- For an easier and less intense position, you can rest on your knees instead of your toes.
- To make the push up more challenging, you can lower your chest towards the plate by bending your elbow.
- To further intensify this exercise, you can rest on one hand on the plate.

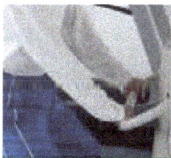

SMALL PUSH UP

Targets: There are two ways of performing small push ups, which are slightly more intense than regular PUSH UP.

- Hold on to the two edges of the plate as shown in the photo.
- More challenging position is to put your hands on the plate touching your thumbs and index fingers together making a heart.

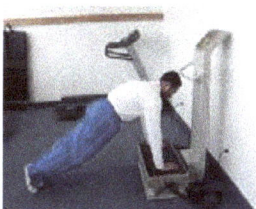

PUSH UP PLUS

Targets: Scapular stabilizers especially, serratus anterior, Chest (pectoralis), shoulders (anterior, lateral and posterior deltoid), biceps, triceps, rhomboids, back and abdominal.

- Assume same position as regular PUSH UP.
- Push your upper back away from your arm or in other words push away from the plate with your arms at the shoulder.

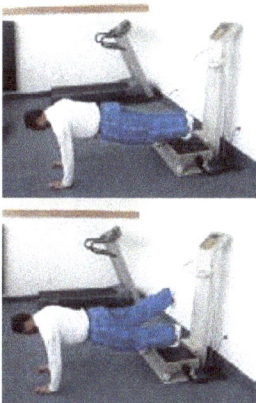

PELVIS STABILIZATION

Targets: Pelvis stabilizers (gluts med_and_max), chest (pectoralis), shoulders (anterior, lateral and posterior deltoid), biceps, triceps, serratus anterior, rhomboids, back and abdominal.

- Assume push up position but with your feet on the plate and hands on the floor.
- Keep your back straight.
- To make this more challenging, lift one leg and hold the position.

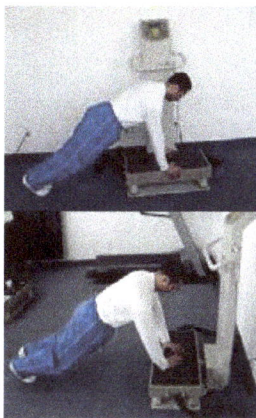

4

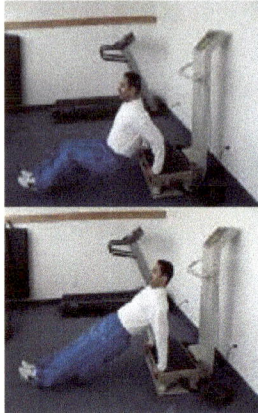

TRICEPS DIP

Targets: Triceps, forearm, posterior shoulder, abdominals, back and gluts.

- Hold on the edge of the plate with your elbows slightly bent.
- For beginners keep the back and the knees slightly bent.
- To intensify the exercise, further bend your elbows.
- To further increase the intensity, straighten your back and knees.
- To make this exercise even more challenging lift one leg and hold the position with your elbows, back and knee straight.

CHAPTER 5

BEGINNERS PROGRAMS

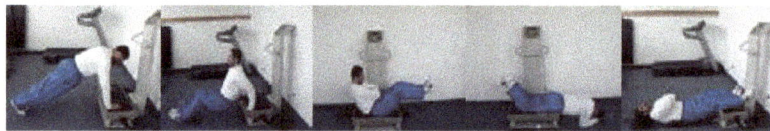

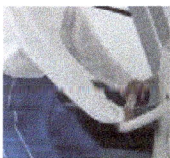

BEGINNERS 1 - 11 MINUTES[66]

MOTION (DIAGRAM) at 20-40 HZ Frequency		HOLD FOR	REST FOR
CALVES		60 SEC	20 SEC
SQUAT		45	
DEEP SQUAT		40	20
LUNGE		Right : 30 Left : 30	10 10
PUSH UP		30	20

5

MOTION (DIAGRAM) at 20-40 HZ Frequency		HOLD FOR	REST FOR
TRICEPS DIP		30 SEC	20 SEC
BASIC ABS		30	20
HAMSTRING STRETCH		45	20
QUADRICEPS MASSAGE		45	20
HAMSTRINGS MASSAGE		45	20
CALVES MASSAGE		45	–

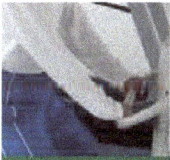

BEGINNERS PROGRAM 2 - 11 MINUTES

	MOTION (DIAGRAM) at 20-40 HZ Frequency	HOLD FOR	REST FOR
CALVES		60 SEC	20 SEC
SQUAT		45	
DEEP SQUAT		40	20
LUNGE		Right : 30 Left : 30	10 10
PUSH UP		30	20

5

MOTION (DIAGRAM) at 20-40 HZ Frequency		HOLD FOR	REST FOR
TRICEPS DIP		30 SEC	20 SEC
BASIC ABS		30	20
HAMSTRING STRETCH		45	20
BACK EXTENSION		45	20
FRONT BRIDGE		45	20
BACK BRIDGE		45	–

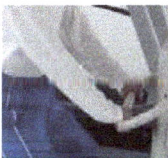

UPPER BODY - 11 MINUTES

MOTION (DIAGRAM) at 20-40 HZ Frequency		HOLD FOR	REST FOR
CALVES		60 SEC	20 SEC
BICEPS CURLS		45	
LATS		45	20
ANTERIOR DELT LATERAL DELT		30 30	10 10
PUSH UP		30	20

5

MOTION (DIAGRAM) at 20-40 HZ Frequency			HOLD FOR	REST FOR
TRICEPS DIP			30 SEC	20 SEC
POSTERIOR DELT			30	20
PEC CROSS			45	20
SHOULDER PRESS			45	20
PUSH UP PLUS			45	20
CALVES MASSAGE			45	

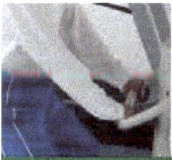

LOWER BODY - 10 MINUTES 25 SEC

MOTION (DIAGRAM) at 20-40 HZ Frequency		HOLD FOR	REST FOR
CALVES		60 sec	20 sec
SQUAT		45	
WIDE STAND SQUAT		60	20
ONE LEGGED STAND		Right: 30 Left: 30	10 30
PELVIC BRIDGE/ BACK BRIDGE		30	30

5

MOTION (DIAGRAM) at 20-40 HZ Frequency	HOLD FOR	REST FOR
SIDE LUNGE	Right: 30 sec Left: 30 sec	10 sec 20 sec
QUADRICEPS MASSAGE	45	20
HAMSTRINGS MASSAGE	45	20
CALVES MASSAGE	45	

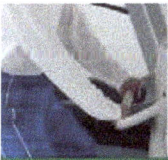

CHAPTER 5

WEIGHT LOSS - 9 MINUTES & 40 SEC

MOTION (DIAGRAM) at 20-40 HZ Frequency	HOLD FOR	REST FOR
CALVES	60 SEC	20 SEC
BASIC ABS	30	20
DIAGONAL CRUNCH	Right: 30 Left: 30	20 20
PELVIS STABILIZATION	30	20
BASIC ABS	30	20
DIAGONAL CRUNCH	Right: 30 Left: 30	20 20

5

MOTION (DIAGRAM) at 20-40 HZ Frequency	HOLD FOR	REST FOR
PELVIS STABILIZATION	30 SEC	20 SEC
QUADRICEPS MASSAGE	60	

CHAPTER 6

BONE DENSITY ENHANCEMENT PROGRAMS

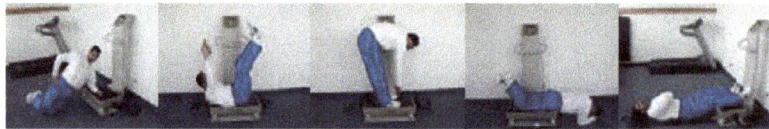

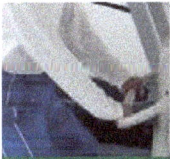

SPINE/BACK BONE DENSITY ENHANCEMENT & CORE - 11 MINUTES

	MOTION (DIAGRAM) at 20-40 HZ Frequency	HOLD FOR	REST FOR
CALVES		60 SEC	20 SEC
FRONT BRIDGE		45	
BACK BRIDGE		45	20
LATERAL RAISE at 15 sec change to other side		Right: 30 Left: 30	10 10
BIRD DOG		30	20

6

MOTION (DIAGRAM) at 20-40 HZ Frequency	HOLD FOR	REST FOR
DEAD BUG	30 SEC	20 SEC
BASIC ABS	30	20
HAMSTRING STRETCH	45	20
QUADRICEPS MASSAGE	45	20
HAMSTRINGS MASSAGE	45	20
CALVES MASSAGE	45	

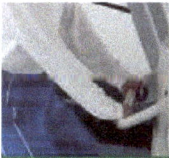

HIP BONE DENSITY ENHANCEMENT - 11 MINUTES

MOTION (DIAGRAM) at 20-40 HZ Frequency		HOLD FOR	REST FOR
CALVES		60 SEC	20 SEC
SQUAT		45	
DEEP SQUAT		45	20
LUNGE		Right: 30 Left: 30	10 10
SQUAT		45	

6

MOTION (DIAGRAM) at 20-40 HZ Frequency	HOLD FOR	REST FOR
DEEP SQUAT	45 SEC	20 SEC
LUNGE	Right: 30 Left: 30	10 10
SQUAT	45	
DEEP SQUAT	45 SEC	20 SEC
LUNGE	Right: 30 Left: 30	10 10

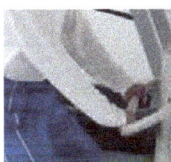

HIP BONE DENSITY ENHANCEMENT - 11 MINUTES

MOTION (DIAGRAM) at 20-40 HZ Frequency		HOLD FOR	REST FOR
HAMSTRING STRETCH		45 SEC	20 SEC
QUADRICEPS MASSAGE		45	20
HAMSTRINGS MASSAGE		45	20
CALVES MASSAGE		45	

6

BONE DENSITY ENHANCEMENT FULL BODY - 19 MINUTES

	MOTION (DIAGRAM) at 20-40 HZ Frequency	HOLD FOR	REST FOR
CALVES		60 SEC	30 SEC
SQUAT		60	
DEEP SQUAT		60	30
WIDE STAND SQUAT		60	30
LUNGE		Right : 60 Left : 60	20 30

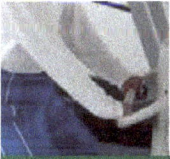

CHAPTER 6

BONE DENSITY ENHANCEMENT FULL BODY - 19 MINUTES

MOTION (DIAGRAM) at 20-40 HZ Frequency		HOLD FOR	REST FOR
FRONT BRIDGE		30 SEC	20 SEC
BACK BRIDGE		30	30
LATERAL RAISE at 15 sec change to other side		30	30
BASIC ABS		30	20
DIAGONAL CRUNCH		Right : 30 Left : 30	20 30

6

MOTION (DIAGRAM) at 20-40 HZ Frequency	HOLD FOR	REST FOR
BIRD DOG	60 SEC	30 SEC
DEAD BUG	60	30
HAMSTRINGS MASSAGE	60	30
CALVES MASSAGE	60	

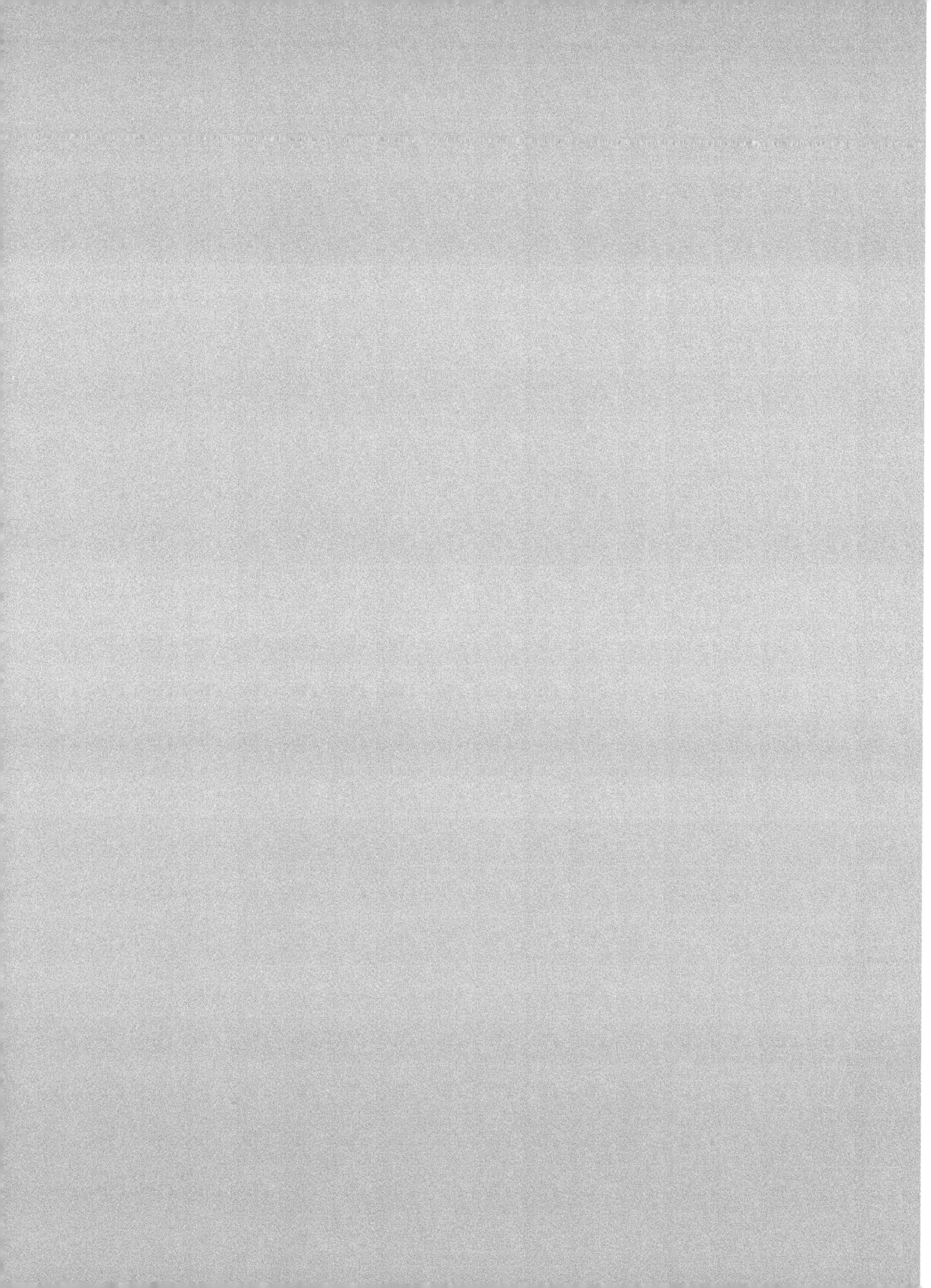

CHAPTER 7

FULL BODY PROGRAMS

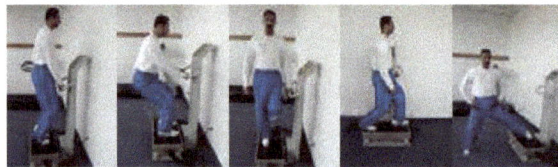

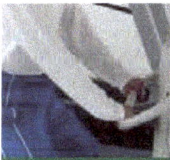

FULL BODY PROGRAMS

PERFORMANCE PROGRAM - 16 MINUTES 40 SEC

MOTION (DIAGRAM) at 20-40 HZ Frequency		HOLD FOR	REST FOR
CALVES		60 SEC	30 SEC
SQUAT		60	
DEEP SQUAT		60	30
WIDE STAND SQUAT		60	30
ONE LEGGED STAND		Right: 30 Left: 30	10 20

7

MOTION (DIAGRAM) at 20-40 HZ Frequency		HOLD FOR	REST FOR
SIDE LUNGE		Right: 30 SEC Left: 30 SEC	10 SEC 10 SEC
CALF STRETCH UP		Right: 30 Left: 30	10 20
ADDUCTOR STRETCH		Right: 30 Left: 30	10 10
HAMSTRING STRETCH		60	30
QUADRICEPS MASSAGE		60	30

PERFORMANCE PROGRAM - 16 MINUTES 40 SEC

MOTION(DIAGRAM) at 20-40 HZ Frequency		HOLD FOR	REST FOR
HAMSTRINGS MASSAGE	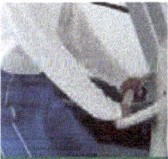	60	30
CALVES MASSAGE		60	

7

ENDURANCE PROGRAM - 19 MINUTES

MOTION(DIAGRAM) at 20-40 HZ Frequency		HOLD FOR	REST FOR
CALVES		60 SEC	30 SEC
SQUAT		60	
DEEP SQUAT		60	30
WIDE STAND SQUAT		60	30
LUNGE		Right : 60 Left : 60	20 30

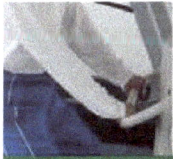

ENDURANCE PROGRAM - 19 MINUTES

MOTION (DIAGRAM) at 20-40 HZ Frequency			HOLD FOR	REST FOR
PUSH UP			30 SEC	20 SEC
PUSH UP SMALL			30	30
TRICEPS DIP			30	30
BASIC ABS			30	20
DIAGONAL CRUNCH			Right : 30 Left : 30	20 20
HAMSTRING STRETCH			60	30

7

MOTION (DIAGRAM) at 20-40 HZ Frequency		HOLD FOR	REST FOR
QUADRICEPS MASSAGE		60 SEC	30 SEC
HAMSTRINGS MASSAGE		60	30
CALVES MASSAGE		60	

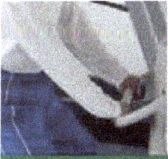

FULL BODY STRENGTHENING - 19 MINUTES

	MOTION (DIAGRAM) at 20-40 HZ Frequency	HOLD FOR	REST FOR
CALVES		60 SEC	30 SEC
SQUAT		60	
DEEP SQUAT		60	30
WIDE STAND SQUAT		60	30
LUNGE		Right : 60 Left : 60	20 30

7

MOTION (DIAGRAM) at 20-40 HZ Frequency	HOLD FOR	REST FOR
FRONT BRIDGE	30 SEC	20 SEC
BACK BRIDGE	30	30
LATERAL RAISE at 15 sec change to other side	30	30
BASIC ABS	30	20
DIAGONAL CRUNCH	Right : 30 Left : 30	20 20

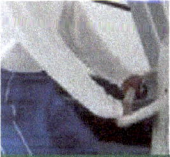

FULL BODY STRENGTHENING - 19 MINUTES

MOTION (DIAGRAM) at 20-40 HZ Frequency		HOLD FOR	REST FOR
BICEPS CURLS		60 SEC	30 SEC
LATS		60	30
LATERAL DELT		60	30
POSTERIOR DELT		60	

7

FULL BODY CORE - 19 MINUTES

MOTION (DIAGRAM) at 20-40 HZ Frequency		HOLD FOR	REST FOR
CALVES		60 SEC	30 SEC
SQUAT		60	
DEEP SQUAT		60	30
WIDE STAND SQUAT		60	30
LUNGE		Right : 60 Left : 60	20 30

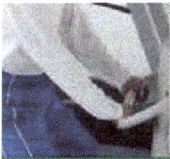

FULL BODY CORE - 19 MINUTES

MOTION (DIAGRAM) at 20-40 HZ Frequency		HOLD FOR	REST FOR
FRONT BRIDGE		30 SEC	20 SEC
BACK BRIDGE		30	30
LATERAL RAISE at 15 sec change to other side		30	30
BASIC ABS		30	20
DIAGONAL CRUNCH		Right : 30 Left : 30	20 20

7

MOTION (DIAGRAM) at 20-40 HZ Frequency	HOLD FOR	REST FOR
BIRD DOG	60 SEC	30 SEC
DEAD BUG	60	30
PUSH UP	60	30
PUSH UP PLUS	60	

CHAPTER 8

SPORTS SPECIFIC PROGRAMS

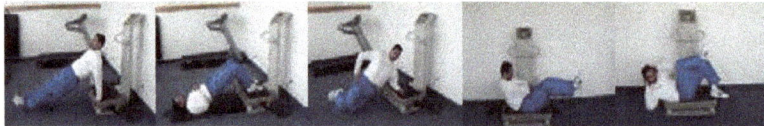

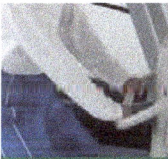

TAEKWONDO/MARTIAL ARTS - 19 MINUTES

MOTION (DIAGRAM) at 20-40 HZ Frequency		HOLD FOR	REST FOR
CALVES		60 SEC	30 SEC
SQUAT		60	
DEEP SQUAT		60	30
WIDE STAND SQUAT		60	30
LUNGE		Right : 60 Left : 60	20 30

8

MOTION (DIAGRAM) at 20-40 HZ Frequency	HOLD FOR	REST FOR
FRONT BRIDGE	30 SEC	20 SEC
BACK BRIDGE	30	30
LATERAL RAISE at 15 sec change to other side	30	30
BASIC ABS	30	20
DIAGONAL CRUNCH	Right : 30 Left : 30	20 20

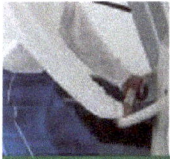

TAEKWONDO/MARTIAL ARTS - 19 MINUTES

MOTION (DIAGRAM) at 20-40 HZ Frequency	HOLD FOR	REST FOR
BIRD DOG	60 SEC	30 SEC
SHOULDER PRESS	60	30
PUSH UP	60	30
PUSH UP PLUS	60	

8

TENNIS/GOLF PROGRAM - 19 MINUTES

	MOTION (DIAGRAM) at 20-40 HZ Frequency	HOLD FOR	REST FOR
CALVES		60 SEC	30 SEC
SQUAT		60	
DEEP SQUAT		60	30
WIDE STAND SQUAT		60	30
LUNGE		Right : 60 Left : 60	20 30

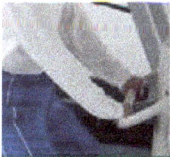

TENNIS/GOLF PROGRAM - 19 MINUTES

	MOTION (DIAGRAM) at 20-40 HZ Frequency	HOLD FOR	REST FOR
FRONT BRIDGE		30 SEC	20 SEC
BACK BRIDGE		30	30
LATERAL RAISE at 15 sec change to other side		30	30
BASIC ABS		30	20
DIAGONAL CRUNCH		Right : 30 Left : 30	20 20

8

MOTION (DIAGRAM) at 20-40 HZ Frequency		HOLD FOR	REST FOR
PUSH UP PLUS		60 SEC	30 SEC
LATS		60	30
SHOULDER PRESS		60	30
POSTERIOR DELT		60	30

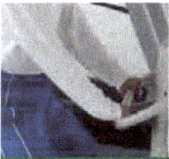

SOCCER - 19 MINUTES

	MOTION (DIAGRAM) at 20-40 HZ Frequency	HOLD FOR	REST FOR
CALVES		60 SEC	30 SEC
SQUAT		60	
DEEP SQUAT		60	30
ONE LEGGED STANCE		30 EACH SIDE	30
LUNGE		Right : 60 Left : 60	20 30

8

MOTION (DIAGRAM) at 20-40 HZ Frequency	HOLD FOR	REST FOR
FRONT BRIDGE	30 SEC	20 SEC
BACK BRIDGE	30	30
LATERAL RAISE at 15 sec change to other side	30	30
BASIC ABS	30	20
DIAGONAL CRUNCH	Right : 30 Left : 30	20 20

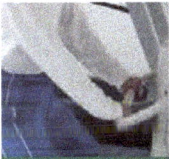

SPORTS SPECIFIC PROGRAMS

SOCCER - 19 MINUTES

MOTION (DIAGRAM) at 20-40 HZ Frequency		HOLD FOR	REST FOR
BIRD DOG		60 SEC	30 SEC
SHOULDER PRESS		60	30
PUSH UP		60	30
PUSH UP PLUS		60	

AMERICAN FOOTBALL - 21 MINUTES

MOTION (DIAGRAM) at 20-40 HZ Frequency		HOLD FOR	REST FOR
CALVES		60 SEC	30 SEC
SQUAT		60	
DEEP SQUAT		60	30
WIDE STAND SQUAT		60	30
LUNGE		Right : 60 Left : 60	20 30

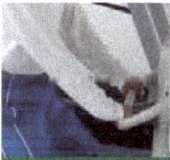

AMERICAN FOOTBALL - 21 MINUTES

MOTION (DIAGRAM) at 20-40 HZ Frequency		HOLD FOR	REST FOR
FRONT BRIDGE		30 SEC	20 SEC
BACK BRIDGE		30	30
LATERAL RAISE at 15 sec change to other side		30	30
BASIC ABS		30	20
DIAGONAL CRUNCH		Right : 30 Left : 30	20 20

8

MOTION (DIAGRAM) at 20-40 HZ Frequency	HOLD FOR	REST FOR
BICEPS CURLS	60 SEC	30 SEC
LATS	60	30
LATERAL DELT	60	20
PEC CROSS	60	20
SHOULDER PRESS	60	30

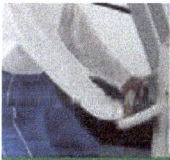

HOCKEY - 21 MINUTES

	MOTION (DIAGRAM) at 20-40 HZ Frequency	HOLD FOR	REST FOR
CALVES		60 SEC	30 SEC
SQUAT		60	
DEEP SQUAT		60	30
WIDE STAND SQUAT		60	30
LUNGE		Right : 60 Left : 60	20 30

8

MOTION (DIAGRAM) at 20-40 HZ Frequency	HOLD FOR	REST FOR
ADDUCTOR STRETCH	Right : 30 SEC Left : 30 SEC	
FRONT BRIDGE	30	20
BACK BRIDGE	30	30
LATERAL RAISE at 15 sec change to other side	30	30
BASIC ABS	30	20

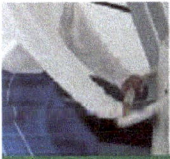

SPORTS SPECIFIC PROGRAMS

HOCKEY - 21 MINUTES

MOTION (DIAGRAM) at 20-40 HZ Frequency		HOLD FOR	REST FOR
DIAGONAL CRUNCH		Right : 30 SEC Left : 30 SEC	20 SEC 20 SEC
BICEPS CURLS		60	30
LATS		60	20
LATERAL DELT		60	20
PEC CROSS		60	20

8

BASEBALL - 21 MINUTES

MOTION (DIAGRAM) at 20-40 HZ Frequency		HOLD FOR	REST FOR
CALVES		60 SEC	30 SEC
SQUAT		60	
DEEP SQUAT		60	30
ONE LEGGED STAND		Right: 30 Left: 30	30
LUNGE		Right: 60 Left: 60	20 30

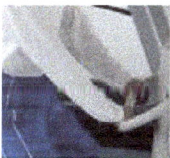

BASEBALL - 21 MINUTES

MOTION (DIAGRAM) at 20-40 HZ Frequency		HOLD FOR	REST FOR
FRONT BRIDGE		30 SEC	20 SEC
BACK BRIDGE		30	30
LATERAL RAISE at 15 sec change to other side		30	30
BASIC ABS		30	20
DIAGONAL CRUNCH		Right : 30 Left : 30	20 20

MOTION (DIAGRAM) at 20-40 HZ Frequency	HOLD FOR	REST FOR
BIRD DOG	60 SEC	30 SEC
SHOULDER PRESS	60	30
PUSH UP	60	30
PUSH UP PLUS	60	
ANTERIOR DELT, LATERAL DELT	30 / 30	10 / 20
POSTERIOR DELT	30	

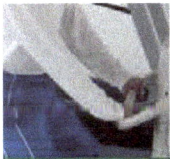

RUNNING - 19 MINUTES

MOTION (DIAGRAM) at 20-40 HZ Frequency	HOLD FOR	REST FOR
CALVES	60 SEC	30 SEC
SQUAT	60	
DEEP SQUAT	60	30
ONE LEGGED STAND	30 EACH SIDE	30
LUNGE	Right : 60 Left : 60	20 30

8

MOTION (DIAGRAM) at 20-40 HZ Frequency		HOLD FOR	REST FOR
FRONT BRIDGE		30 SEC	20 SEC
BACK BRIDGE		30	30
LATERAL RAISE at 15 sec change to other side		30	30
BASIC ABS		30	20
DIAGONAL CRUNCH		Right : 30 Left : 30	20 20

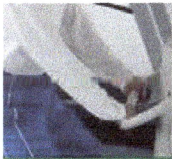

CHAPTER 8

RUNNING - 19 MINUTES

MOTION (DIAGRAM) at 20-40 HZ Frequency			HOLD FOR	REST FOR
BIRD DOG			60 SEC	30 SEC
SHOULDER PRESS			60	30
PUSH UP			60	30
PUSH UP PLUS			60	

8

SWIMMING - 21 MINUTES

MOTION (DIAGRAM) at 20-40 HZ Frequency	HOLD FOR	REST FOR
CALVES	60 SEC	30 SEC
SQUAT	60	
DEEP SQUAT	60	30
LUNGE	Right : 60 Left : 60	20 30
FRONT BRIDGE	30	20

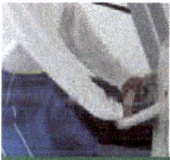

SWIMMING - 21 MINUTES

MOTION (DIAGRAM) at 20-40 HZ Frequency		HOLD FOR	REST FOR
BACK BRIDGE		30 SEC	30 SEC
LATERAL RAISE at 15 sec change to other side		30	30
BASIC ABS		30	20
DIAGONAL CRUNCH		Right : 30 Left : 30	20 20
BIRD DOG		60	30

8

MOTION (DIAGRAM) at 20-40 HZ Frequency	HOLD FOR	REST FOR
SHOULDER PRESS	60 SEC	30 SEC
PUSH UP	60	30
PUSH UP PLUS	60	
LATS	60	20
ANTERIOR DELT, LATERAL DELT	30 / 30	10 / 20
POSTERIOR DELT	30	

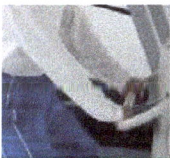

VOLLEYBALL - 21 MINUTES

MOTION (DIAGRAM) at 20-40 HZ Frequency		HOLD FOR	REST FOR
CALVES		60 SEC	30 SEC
SQUAT		60	
DEEP SQUAT		60	30
LUNGE		Right : 60 Left : 60	20 30
FRONT BRIDGE		30	20

8

MOTION (DIAGRAM) at 20-40 HZ Frequency	HOLD FOR	REST FOR
BACK BRIDGE	30 SEC	30 SEC
LATERAL RAISE at 15 sec change to other side	30	30
BASIC ABS	30	20
DIAGONAL CRUNCH	Right : 30 Left : 30	20 20
BIRD DOG	60	30

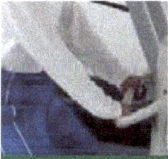

VOLLEYBALL - 21 MINUTES

MOTION (DIAGRAM) at 20-40 HZ Frequency		HOLD FOR	REST FOR
SHOULDER PRESS		60 SEC	30 SEC
PUSH UP		60	30
PUSH UP PLUS		60	
BICEPS CURLS		60	30
ANTERIOR DELT, LATERAL DELT		30 / 30	10 / 20
POSTERIOR DELT		30	

8

BIKING - 16 MINUTES

MOTION (DIAGRAM) at 20-40 HZ Frequency	HOLD FOR	REST FOR
CALVES	60 SEC	30 SEC
SQUAT	60	
DEEP SQUAT	60	30
LUNGE	Right : 60 Left : 60	20 30
FRONT BRIDGE	30	20

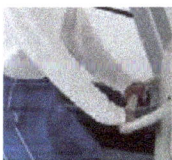

BIKING - 16 MINUTES

MOTION (DIAGRAM) at 20-40 HZ Frequency		HOLD FOR	REST FOR
BACK BRIDGE		30 SEC	30 SEC
LATERAL RAISE at 15 sec change to other side		30	30
BASIC ABS		30	20
DIAGONAL CRUNCH		Right : 30 Left : 30	20 20
BIRD DOG		60	30

8

MOTION (DIAGRAM) at 20-40 HZ Frequency		HOLD FOR	REST FOR
PUSH UP		60	30
PUSH UP PLUS		60	

CHAPTER 9

HIGH INTENSITY BOOTCAMP PROGRAMS

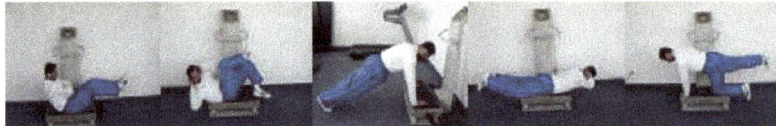

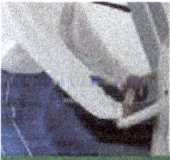

CHAPTER 9

QUICK 4 - 4 MINUTES 30 SEC - NO REST

MOTION (DIAGRAM) at 20-40 HZ Frequency		ACTIVE TIME
CALVES		30 SEC
SQUAT		30
DEEP SQUAT		30
BASIC ABS		30
DIAGONAL CRUNCH		Right : 30 Left : 30

9

MOTION (DIAGRAM) at 20-40 HZ Frequency	ACTIVE TIME
PUSH UP	30 SEC
TRICEPS DIP	30
BACK EXTENSION	30

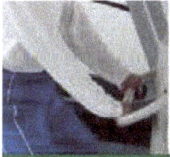

QUICK 12 - HIGH INTENSITY 12 MINUTES BOOTCAMP PROGRAM

MOTION (DIAGRAM) @ 20-35 HZ FREQUENCY		HOLD FOR
CALVES		60 SEC
DEEP SQUAT		60
SIDE LUNGES		30 SEC EACH
PUSH UP PLUS		30
SHOULDER PRESS		30

9

MOTION (DIAGRAM) @ 20-35 HZ FREQUENCY		HOLD FOR
TRICEPS DIP		30 SEC
LATERAL RAISE		30 SEC EACH
BASIC ABS		30
DIAGONAL CRUNCH		30 SEC EACH
DEAD BUG		60 SEC EACH
BIRD DOG		30 SEC EACH

HIGH INTESITY 12 MINUTES BOOTCAMP PROGRAM

MOTION (DIAGRAM) @ 20-35 HZ FREQUENCY		HOLD FOR
BACK EXTENSION	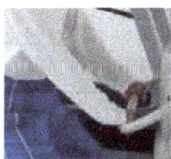	30
BACK BRIDGE		60

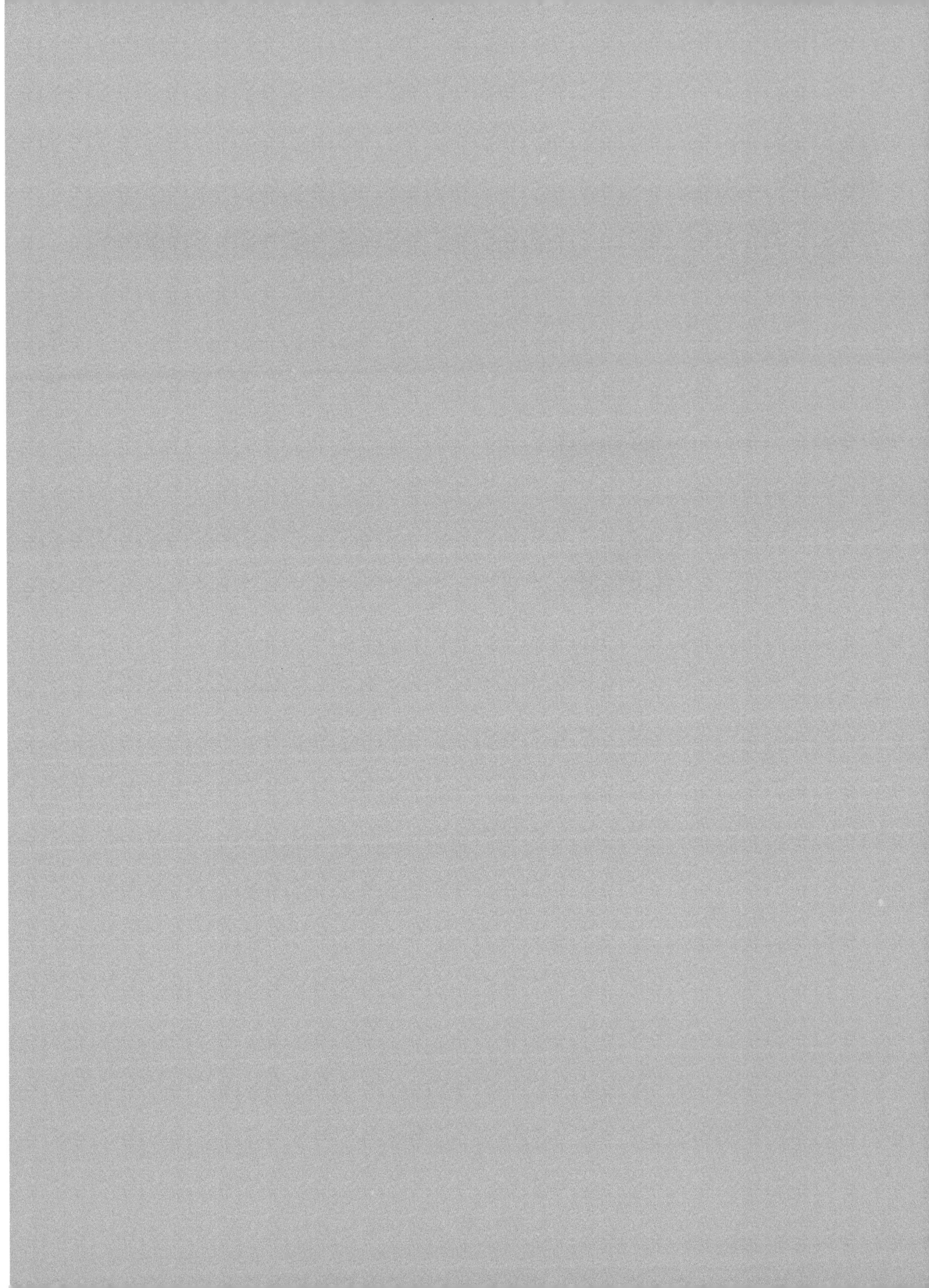

CHAPTER 10
PROGRAM SUMMARY TABLES

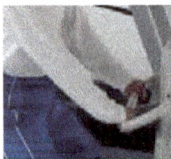

BEGINNERS 1. 11 MINUTES

A quick training session designed for those who haven't been training for a while!!

MOTION (DIAGRAM) at 20-40 HZ Frequency	HOLD FOR	REST FOR
CALVES	60 SEC	20 SEC
SQUAT	45	
DEEP SQUAT	45	20
LUNGE	Right: 30 / Left: 30	10 / 10
PUSH UP	30	20
TRICEPS DIP	30	20
BASIC ABS	30	20
HAMSTRING STRETCH	45	20
QUADRICEPS MASSAGE	45	20
HAMSTRINGS MASSAGE	45	20
CALVES MASSAGE	45	

BEGINNERS 2 - 11 MINUTES

MOTION (DIAGRAM) at 20-40 HZ Frequency	HOLD FOR	REST FOR
CALVES	60 SEC	20 SEC
SQUAT	45	
DEEP SQUAT	45	20
LUNGE	Right: 30 / Left: 30	10 / 10
PUSH UP	30	20
TRICEPS DIP	30	20
BASIC ABS	30	20
HAMSTRING STRETCH	45	20
BACK EXTENSION	45	20
FRONT BRIDGE	45	20
BACK BRIDGE	45	

UPPER BODY - 11 MINUTES

MOTION (DIAGRAM) at 20-40 HZ Frequency	HOLD FOR	REST FOR
CALVES	60 SEC	20 SEC
BICEPS CURLS	45	
LATS	45	20
ANTERIOR DELT / LATERAL DELT	Right: 30 / Left: 30	10 / 10
PUSH UP	30	20
TRICEPS DIP	30	20
POSTERIOR DELT	30	20
PEC CROSS	45	20
SHOULDER PRESS	45	20
PUSH UP PLUS	45	20
CALVES MASSAGE	45	

10

LOWER BODY - 10 MINUTES 25 SEC

MOTION (DIAGRAM) at 20-35 HZ FREQUENCY	HOLD FOR	REST FOR
CALVES	60 SEC	20 SEC
SQUAT	45	
WIDE STANCE SQUAT	60	20
ONE LEGGED STAND	Right: 30 / Left: 30	10 / 30
PELVIC BRIDGE	30	30
SIDE LUNGE	Right: 30 / Left: 30	10 / 20
QUADRICEPS MASSAGE	45	20
HAMSTRINGS MASSAGE	45	20
CALVES MASSAGE	45	

SPINE/BACK BONE DENSITY ENHANCEMENT & CORE - 11 MINUTES

MOTION (DIAGRAM) at 20-40 HZ Frequency	HOLD FOR	REST FOR
CALVES	60 SEC	20 SFC
SQUAT	45	
DEEP SQUAT	45	20
LUNGE	Right: 30 / Left: 30	10 / 10
SQUAT	45	
DEEP SQUAT	45	20 / 10
LUNGE	Right: 30 / Left: 30	10
HAMSTRING STRETCH	45	20
QUADRICEPS MASSAGE	45	20
HAMSTRINGS MASSAGE	45	20
CALVES MASSAGE	45	

HIP BONE DENSITY ENHANCEMENT - 11 MINUTES

MOTION (DIAGRAM) at 20-40 HZ Frequency	HOLD FOR	REST FOR
CALVES	60 SEC	20 SEC
FRONT BRIDGE	45	
BACK BRIDGE	45	20
LATERAL RAISE	Right: 30 / Left: 30	10 / 10
BIRD DOG	30	20
DEAD BUG	30	20
BASIC ABS	30	20
HAMSTRING STRETCH	45	20
QUADRICEPS MASSAGE	45	20
HAMSTRINGS MASSAGE	45	20
CALVES MASSAGE	45	
CALVES MASSAGE	45	

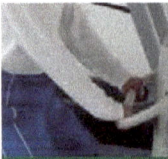

FULL BODY BONE DENSITY ENHANCEMENT - 19 MINUTES

MOTION (DIAGRAM) @ 20-35 HZ FREQUENCY	HOLD FOR	REST FOR
CALVES	60 SEC	30 SEC
SQUAT	60	
DEEP SQUAT	60	30
WIDE STAND SQUAT	60	30
LUNGE	Right: 60 / Left: 60	20 / 30
FRONT BRIDGE	30	20
BACK BRIDGE	30	30
LATERAL RAISE at 15 sec change to other side	30	30
BASIC ABS	30	20
DIAGONAL CRUNCH	Right: 30 / Left: 30	20 / 20
BIRD DOG	60	30
DEAD BUG	60	30
HAMSTRINGS MASSAGE	60	30
CALVES MASSAGE	60	

PERFORMANCE - 16 MINUTES 40 SEC

MOTION (DIAGRAM) @ 20-35 HZ FREQUENCY	HOLD FOR	REST FOR
CALVES	60 SEC	30 SEC
SQUAT	60	
DEEP SQUAT	60	30
WIDE STAND SQUAT	60	30
ONE LEGGED STAND	Right: 30 / Left: 30	10 / 20
SIDE LUNGE	Right: 30 / Left: 30	10 / 10
CALF STRETCH UP	Right: 30 / Left: 30	10 / 20
ADDUCTOR STRETCH	Right: 30 / Left: 30	10 / 10
HAMSTRING STRETCH	60	30
QUADRICEPS MASSAGE	60	30
HAMSTRINGS MASSAGE	60	30
CALVES MASSAGE	60	

Increase your muscle power. Particularly beneficial for athletes who want that extra performance edge. Beginner to advanced.

ENDURANCE - 19 MINUTES

Improve cardiovascular endurance. Ideal for training for sports that require strong cardiovascular output.

MOTION (DIAGRAM) @ 20-35 HZ FREQUENCY	HOLD FOR	REST FOR
CALVES	60 SEC	30 SEC
SQUAT	60	
DEEP SQUAT	60	30
WIDE STAND SQUAT	60	30
LUNGE	Right: 60 / Left: 60	20 / 30
PUSH UP	30	20
PUSH UP SMALL	30	30
TRICEPS DIP	30	30
BASIC ABS	30	20
DIAGNOAL CRUNCH	Right: 30 / Left: 30	20 / 20
HAMSTRING STRETCH	60	30
QUADRICEPS MASSAGE	60	30
HAMSTRINGS MASSAGE	60	30
CALVES MASSAGE	60	

FULL BODY CORE - 19 MINUTES

MOTION (DIAGRAM) @ 20-35 HZ FREQUENCY	HOLD FOR	REST FOR
CALVES	60 SEC	60 SEC
SQUAT	60	60
DEEP SQUAT	60	60
WIDE STAND SQUAT	60	60
LUNGE	Right: 60 / Left: 60	Right: 60 / Left: 60
FRONT BRIDGE	30	30
BACK BRIDGE	30	30
LATERAL RAISE at 15 sec change to other side	30	30
BASIC ABS	30	30
DIAGONAL CRUNCH	Right: 30 / Left: 30	Right: 30 / Left: 30
BIRD DOG	60	60
DEAD BUG	60	60
PUSH UP	60	60
PUSH UP PLUS	60	60

FULL BODY STRENGTHENING - 19 MINUTES

MOTION (DIAGRAM) @ 20-35 HZ FREQUENCY	HOLD FOR	REST FOR
CALVES	60 SEC	30 SEC
SQUAT	60	
DEEP SQUAT	60	30
WIDE STAND SQUAT	60	30
LUNGE	Right: 60 / Left: 60	20 / 30
FRONT BRIDGE	30	20
BACK BRIDGE	30	30
LATERAL RAISE at 15 sec change to other side	30	30
BASIC ABS	30	20
DIAGNOAL CRUNCH	Right: 30 / Left: 30	20 / 20
BICEPS CURLS	60	30
LATS	60	30
LATERAL DELT	60	30
POSTERIOR SHOULDER	60	

WEIGHT LOSS PROGRAM - 9 MINUTES & 40 SEC

Tone muscles and lose inches off your abdomen, waist, upper arms and thighs. Best for beginners.

MOTION (DIAGRAM) @ 20-35 HZ FREQUENCY	HOLD FOR	REST FOR
CALVES	60 SEC	20 SEC
BASIC ABS	30	20
DIAGNAL CRUNCH	Right: 30 / Left: 30	20 / 20
PELVIS STABILIZATION	30	20
BASIC ABS	30	20
DIAGNOAL CRUNCH	Right: 30 / Left: 30	20 / 20
PELVIS STABILIZATION	30	20
QUADRICEPS MASSAGE	60	

Say good bye to those pounds- with no sweat or tears! WBV technology and programming will do all the work for you.
The easy way to slim down!!

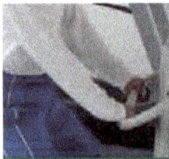

TAEKWONDO/MARTIAL ARTS - 19 MINUTES

MOTION (DIAGRAM) @ 20-35 HZ FREQUENCY	HOLD FOR	REST FOR
CALVES	60 SEC	30 SEC
SQUAT	60	
DEEP SQUAT	60	30
WIDE STAND SQUAT	60	30
LUNGE	Right: 60 / Left: 60	20 / 30
FRONT BRIDGE	30	20
BACK BRIDGE	30	30
LATERAL RAISE at 15 sec change to other side	30	30
BASIC ABS	30	20
DIAGONAL CRUNCH	Right: 30 / Left: 30	20 / 20
PUSH UP PLUS	60	30
LATS	60	30
SHOULDER PRESS	60	30
POSTERIOR SHOULDER	60	

TENNIS/GOLF PROGRAM - 19 MINUTES

MOTION (DIAGRAM) @ 20-35 HZ FREQUENCY	HOLD FOR	REST FOR
CALVES	60 SEC	30 SEC
SQUAT	60	
DEEP SQUAT	60	30
WIDE STAND SQUAT	60	30
LUNGE	Right: 60 / Left: 60	20 / 30
FRONT BRIDGE	30	20
BACK BRIDGE	30	30
LATERAL RAISE at 15 sec change to other side	30	30
BASIC ABS	30	20
DIAGONAL CRUNCH	Right: 30 / Left: 30	20 / 20
BIRD DOG	60	30
SHOULDER PRESS	60	30
PUSH UP	60	30
PUSH UP PLUS	60	

SOCCER - 19 MINUTES

MOTION (DIAGRAM) @ 20-40 HZ FREQUENCY	HOLD FOR	REST FOR
CALVES	60 SEC	30 SEC
SQUAT	60	
DEEP SQUAT	60	30
ONE LEGGED STANCE	30 each side	30
LUNGE	Right: 60 / Left: 60	20 / 30
FRONT BRIDGE	30	20
BACK BRIDGE	30	30
LATERAL RAISE at 15 sec change to other side	30	30
BASIC ABS	30	20
DIAGONAL CRUNCH	Right: 30 / Left: 30	20 / 20
BIRD DOG	60	30
SHOULDER PRESS	60	30
PUSH UP	60	30
PUSH UP PLUS	60	

10

AMERCAN FOOTBALL - 21 MINUTES

MOTION (DIAGRAM) @ 20-40 HZ FREQUENCY	HOLD FOR	REST FOR
CALVES	60 SEC	30 SEC
SQUAT	60	
DEEP SQUAT	60	30
WIDE STAND SQUAT	60	30
LUNGE	Right: 60 / Left: 60	20 / 30
FRONT BRIDGE	30	20
BACK BRIDGE	30	30
LATERAL RAISE at 15 sec change to other side	30	30
BASIC ABS	30	20
DIAGONAL CRUNCH	Right: 30 / Left: 30	20 / 20
BICEPS CURLS	60	30
LATS	60	20
LATERAL DELT	60	20
PEC CROSS	60	20
SHOULDER PRESS	60	

HOCKEY - 21 MINUTES

MOTION (DIAGRAM) @ 20-40 HZ FREQUENCY	HOLD FOR	REST FOR
CALVES	60 SEC	30 SEC
SQUAT	60	
DEEP SQUAT	60	30
WIDE STAND SQUAT	60	30
LUNGE	Right: 60 / Left: 60	20 / 30
ADDUCTOR STRETCH	Right: 30 / Left: 30	
FRONT BRIDGE	30	20
BACK BRIDGE	30	30
LATERAL RAISE at 15 sec change to other side	30	30
BASIC ABS	30	20
DIAGONAL CRUNCH	Right: 30 / Left: 30	20 / 20
BICEPS CURLS	60	30
LATS	60	20
LATERAL DELT	60	20
PEC CROSS	60	20

BASEBALL - 21 MINUTES

MOTION (DIAGRAM) @ 20-40 HZ FREQUENCY	HOLD FOR	REST FOR
CALVES	60 SEC	30 SEC
SQUAT	60	
DEEP SQUAT	60	30
ONE LEGGED STANCE	Right: 30 / Left: 30	30
LUNGE	Right: 60 / Left: 60	20 / 30
FRONT BRIDGE	30	20
BACK BRIDGE	30	30
LATERAL RAISE at 15 sec change to other side	30	30
BASIC ABS	30	20
DIAGONAL CRUNCH	Right: 30 / Left: 30	20 / 20
BIRD DOG	60	30
SHOULDER PRESS	60	30
PUSH UP	60	30
PUSH UP PLUS	60	
ANTERIOR, LATERAL DELT	30/30	10/20
POSTERIOR DELT	30	

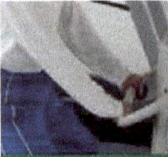

RUNNING - 19 MINUTES

MOTION (DIAGRAM) @ 20-40 HZ FREQUENCY	HOLD FOR	REST FOR
CALVES	60 SEC	30 SEC
SQUAT	60	
DEEP SQUAT	60	30
ONE LEGGED STANCE	30 each side	30
LUNGE	Right: 60 / Left: 60	20 / 30
FRONT BRIDGE	30	20
BACK BRIDGE	30	30
LATERAL RAISE at 15 sec change to other side	30	30
BASIC ABS	30	20
DIAGONAL CRUNCH	Right: 30 / Left: 30	20 / 20
BIRD DOG	60	30
SHOULDER PRESS	60	30
PUSH UP	60	30
PUSH UP PLUS	60	

SWIMMING - 21 MINUTES

MOTION (DIAGRAM) @ 20-40 HZ FREQUENCY	HOLD FOR	REST FOR
CALVES	60 SEC	30 SEC
SQUAT	60	
DEEP SQUAT	60	30
LUNGE	Right: 60 / Left: 60	20 / 30
FRONT BRIDGE	30	20
BACK BRIDGE	30	30
LATERAL RAISE at 15 sec change to other side	30	30
BASIC ABS	30	20
DIAGONAL CRUNCH	Right: 30 / Left: 30	20 / 20
BIRD DOG	60	30
SHOULDER PRESS	60	30
PUSH UP	60	30
PUSH UP PLUS	60	
LATS	60	20
ANTERIOR DELT, LATERAL DELT	30/30	10/20
POSTERIOR DELT	30	

VOLLEYBALL - 21 MINUTES

MOTION (DIAGRAM) @ 20-40 HZ FREQUENCY	HOLD FOR	REST FOR
CALVES	60 SEC	30 SEC
SQUAT	60	
DEEP SQUAT	60	30
LUNGE	Right: 60 / Left: 60	20 / 30
FRONT BRIDGE	30	20
BACK BRIDGE	30	30
LATERAL RAISE at 15 sec change to other side	30	30
BASIC ABS	30	20
DIAGONAL CRUNCH	Right: 30 / Left: 30	20 / 20
BIRD DOG	60	30
SHOULDER PRESS	60	30
PUSH UP	60	30
PUSH UP PLUS	60	
BICEPS CURLS	60	30
ANTERIOR DELT, LATERAL DELT	30/30	10/20
POSTERIOR DELT	30	

10

BIKING - 16 MINUTES

MOTION (DIAGRAM) @ 20-40 HZ FREQUENCY	HOLD FOR	REST FOR
CALVES	60 SEC	30 SEC
SQUAT	60	
DEEP SQUAT	60	30
LUNGE	Right: 60 / Left: 60	20 / 30
FRONT BRIDGE	30	20
BACK BRIDGE	30	30
LATERAL RAISE at 15 sec change to other side	30	30
BASIC ABS	30	20
DIAGONAL CRUNCH	Right: 30 / Left: 30	20 / 20
BIRD DOG	60	30
PUSH UP	60	30
PUSH UP PLUS	60	

QUICK 4 - 4 MINUTES 30 SEC- NO REST

The most effective full body workout in the shortest amount of time. Targets your strength, cardiovascular and flexibility systems in 4 minutes per session!!

MOTION (DIAGRAM) @ 20-35 HZ FREQUENCY	HOLD FOR
CALVES	30 SEC
SQUAT	30
DEEP SQUAT	30
BASIC ABS	30
DIAGONAL CRUNCH	Right: 30 / Left: 30
PUSH UP	30
TRICEPS DIP	30
BACK EXTENSION	30

HIGH INTESITY 12 MINUTES BOOTCAMP PROGRAM

MOTION (DIAGRAM) @ 20-35 HZ FREQUENCY	HOLD FOR
CALVES	60 SEC
DEEP SQUAT	60 SEC
SIDE LUNGES	30 SEC EACH
PUSH UP PLUS	30
SHOUDER PRESS	30
TRICEPS DIP	30
LATERAL RAISE	30 SEC EACH
BASIC ABS	30
DIAGONAL CRUNCH	30 SEC EACH
DEAD BUG	60 SEC EACH
BIRD DOG	30 SEC EACH
BACK EXTENSION	30
BACK BRIDGE	60 SEC

Frequently Asked Questions

Q. What is Whole Body Vibration (WBV) training?
A. WBV training is achieved through holding specific positions on an oscillating platform with a frequency of 5 to 50 Hz. However, research indicates that a frequency of 18 to 35 has the best result. In addition, this oscillation has to be vertical to provide the positive effects.

Q. How does it work?
A. WBV trainer induces vibration that transmits through muscles, bones and soft tissues. Each muscle in order to do its job of holding specific postures has to overcome the vibration first and then hold the position. Research shows to do this 95% of the muscle fibers have to fire. In addition, since the vibration transmits through the whole body there is no escape for all other muscles, bones and soft tissues of the body from the effect of vibration. Therefore, as a natural response they are all activated. This activation counts for overall increased metabolism, strength, power, endurance, bone density, Growth Hormones (fountain of youth, elixir of life), testosterone (increase energy and reproduction), Serotonin and Dopamine (Happy Hormones), blood circulation (increase healing and metabolism), lymphatic drainage (removal of toxins and rejuvenating tissues) and neuromuscular enhancement (increase strength and power) and decreased body fat.

Q. How old is this technology?
A. WBV exercise programs are based on 30 years of research. Whole Body Vibration (WBV) was initially used in Europe in the late 1800's for exercise and therapeutic purposes.

Q. Who has used this training in the past?
A. Whole Body Vibration has been used to treat bone and lean muscle mass loss in astronomers who spend considerable time in space. Many famous actors and singers such as Madonna have used this training to maximize their physics and strength. Most professional football, basketball and hockey teams have been using WBV.

Q. What kind of machine should I purchase?
A. Look for a machine with a vibration frequency of 20 to 45 Hz. Even though some machine offer up to 60 Hz, most research have used equipment with 20-35 Hz and a smaller number have used those with up to 45 Hz.
Ensure that the plate is a generous size. A big plate offers more exercise choices.
Go with a reliable brand. Be sure the warranty and service options are fair and that the company has established a good reputation in the industry.

Q. How long is each session?
A. Based on your goal each session could be from 4 to 20 minutes long. 10 minutes of exercises on WBV trainer is equal to 30-40 minutes of weight training. This makes WBV Exercise programs ideal for busy people who desire to keep active but do not have enough time.

Q. What are the benefits of WBV training?
A. Overall increased metabolism, strength, power, endurance, bone density, Growth Hormones (fountain of youth, elixir of life), testosterone (increase energy and reproduction), Serotonin and Dopamine (Happy Hormones), blood circulation (increase healing and metabolism), lymphatic drainage (removal of toxins and rejuvenating tissues) and neuromuscular enhancement (increase strength and power), and decreased body fat,.

Q. Is WBV training suitable for elderly?
A. WBV program with its soft nature exercise, enhancing balance, hormones and bone density, is the perfect exercise for elderly who desire to increase their strength, balance, bone density and overall wellness. WBV is the only exercise shown recently to increase bone density in post-menopausal women 60-70 years old.

Q. Is WBV training beneficial to athletes?
A. Competitive Athletes will gain the edge that they need to win in strength, power, endurance and overall performance participating in the WBV programs presented in this book.

Q. What kind of programs do you offer in this book?
A. Specific WBV programs are designed and presented in this book to help you achieve your goals, from increasing your bone density, losing weight, strengthening your core to specifically focusing and strengthening your upper or lower limbs.

References

1. Adams JB, Edwards D, Serviette D, Bedient AM, Huntsman E, Jacobs KA, Del Rossi G, Roos BA, Signorile JF. Optimal frequency, displacement, duration, and recovery patterns to maximize power output following acute whole-body vibration. J Strength Cond Res. 2009 Jan;23(1):237-45.

2. Ahlborg L, Andersson C, Julin P. Whole-body vibration training compared with resistance training: effect on spasticity, muscle strength and motor performance in adults with cerebral palsy. J Rehabil Med. 2006 Sep;38(5):302-8.

3. Alentorn-Geli E, Padilla J, Moras G, Lazaro Haro C, Fernandez-Sola J. Six weeks of whole-body vibration exercise improves pain and fatigue in women with fibromyalgia. J Altern Complement Med. 2008 Oct;14(8):975-81.

4. Aleyaasin M, Harrigan JJ. Vibration exercise for treatment of osteoporosis: a theoretical model. Proc Inst Mech Eng [H]. 2008 Oct;222(7):1161-6.

5. Annino G, Padua E, Castagna C, Di Salvo V, Minichella S, Tsarpela O, Manzi V, D'Ottavio S. Effect of whole body vibration training on lower limb performance in selected high-level ballet students. J Strength Cond Res. 2007 Nov;21(4):1072-6.

6. Bakhtiary AH, Safavi-Farokhi Z, Aminian-Far A. Influence of vibration on delayed onset of muscle soreness following eccentric exercise. Br J Sports Med. 2007 Mar;41(3):145-8. Epub 2006 Nov 30.

7. Baum K, Votteler T, Schiab J. Efficiency of vibration exercise for glycemic control in type 2 diabetes patients. Int J Med Sci. 2007 May 31;4(3):159-63.

8. Belavy DL, Hides JA, Wilson SJ, Stanton W, Dimeo FC, Rittweger J, Felsenberg D, Richardson CA. Resistive simulated weightbearing exercise with whole body vibration reduces lumbar spine deconditioning in bed-rest. Spine. 2008 Mar 1;33(5):E121-31.

9. Bogaerts A, Delecluse C, Claessens AL, Coudyzer W, Boonen S, Verschueren SM. Impact of whole-body vibration training versus fitness training on muscle strength and muscle mass in older men: a 1-year randomized controlled trial. J Gerontol A Biol Sci Med Sci. 2007 Jun;62(6):630-5.

10. Bogaerts A, Verschueren S, Delecluse C, Claessens AL, Boonen S. Effects of whole body vibration training on postural control in older individuals: a 1 year randomized controlled trial. Gait Posture. 2007 Jul;26(2):309-16. Epub 2006 Oct 30.

11. Bosco C, Cardinale M, Tsarpela O, Lacatelli E. New trends in training science: the use of vibrations for enhancing performance. European Journal of Applied Physiology 1984. 53: 275-284.

12. Bosco C, Colli R, Introni E, Cardinale M, Iacovelli M, tihanyi J, von Duvillard S, Viru A. Adaptive responses of human skeletal muscle to vibration exposure. Clinical Physiology 1999; 19(2): 4-13.

13. Bosco C, Iacovelli M, Tasarpela O. Hormonal response to whole body vibration in men. Eur J Appl Physiol 2000; 81: 449-452.

14. Bullock N, Martin DT, Ross A, Rosemond CD, Jordan MJ, Marino FE. Acute effect of whole-body vibration on sprint and jumping performance in elite skeleton athletes. J Strength Cond Res. 2008 Jul;22(4):1371-4.

15. Burke J, Schutten M, Koceja D, Kamen E. Age-dependent effects of muscle vibration and the Jendrassik maneuver on the patellar tendon reflex response. Arch. Phys. Med. Rehabil 1996; 77(6): 600-604.

16. Calvisi V, Angelozzi M, Franco A, Mottola L, Crisostomi S, Corsica C, Ferrari M, Quaresima V. Influence of whole-body vibration static exercise on quadriceps oxygenation. Adv Exp Med Biol. 2006;578:137-41. No abstract available.

17. Cardinale M, Erskine JA. Vibration training in elite sport: effective training solution or just another fad? Int J Sports Physiol Perform. 2008 Jun;3(2):232-9.

18. Cardinale M, Leiper J, Farajian P, Heer M. Whole-body vibration can reduce calciuria induced by high protein intakes and may counteract bone resorption: A preliminary study. J Sports Sci. 2007 Jan 1;25(1):111-9.

19. Cardinale M, Soiza RL, Leiper JB, Gibson A, Primrose WR. Hormonal responses to a single session of whole body vibration exercise in elderly individuals. Br J Sports Med. 2008 Apr 15. [Epub ahead of print]

20. Cardinale M, Wakeling J. Whole body vibration exercise: are vibrations good for you?.
British Journal of Sports Medicine 2005; 39:585-589.

21. Carter N, Kannus P, Kahn K. Exercise in the prevention of falls in older people. Sports Med 2001; 31: 427-438.

22. Cheung WH, Mok HW, Qin L, Sze PC, Lee KM, Leung KS. High-frequency whole-body vibration improves balancing ability in elderly women. Arch Phys Med Rehabil. 2007 Jul;88(7):852-7.

23. Cochrane DJ, Sartor F, Winwood K, Stannard SR, Narici MV, Rittweger J. A comparison of the physiologic effects of acute whole-body vibration exercise in young and older people.
Arch Phys Med Rehabil. 2008 May;89(5):815-21.

24. Cochrane DJ, Stannard SR, Sargeant AJ, Rittweger J. The rate of muscle temperature increase during acute whole-body vibration exercise. Eur J Appl Physiol. 2008 Jul;103(4):441-8.

25. Colin L, Eakin M. Knee Arthrofibrosis prevention and management of a potentially devastating condition. The physician and sports medicine 2001; 29(3).

26. Da Silva ME, Fernandez JM, Castillo E, Nunez VM, Vaamonde DM, Poblador MS, Lancho JL. Influence of vibration training on energy expenditure in active men. J Strength Cond Res. 2007 May;21(2):470-5.

27. Delecluse C, Roelants M, Diels R, Koninckx E, Verschueren S. Effects of whole body vibration training on muscle strength and sprint performance in sprint-trained athletes. Int J Sports Med. 2005 Oct;26(8):662-8.

28. Delecluse C, Roelants M, Verschueren S. Strength increase after whole body vibration compared with resistance training. Medicine and Science in Sports and Exercise 2003; 35: 1033-1004.

29. Dolny DG, Reyes GF. Whole body vibration exercise: training and benefits.
Curr Sports Med Rep. 2008 May-Jun;7(3):152-7.

30. Edge J, Mundel T, Weir K, Cochrane DJ. The effects of acute whole body vibration as a recovery modality following high-intensity interval training in well-trained, middle-aged runners.
Eur J Appl Physiol. 2009 Feb;105(3):421-8. Epub 2008 Nov 15.

31. Falempin M, Fodili In-Albon S. Influence of brief daily tendon vibration on rats soleus muscle in non-weight-bearing situation. Journal of applied physiology 1999; 87(1): 3-9.

32. Flieger J, Karachalios T, Khaldi P, Lyritis G. Mechanical stimulation in the form of vibration prevents postmenopausal bone loss in ovariectomized rats. Calcif Tissue Int 1998; 63: 510-515.

33. Gilsanz V, Wren TA, Sanchez M, Dorey F, Judex S, Rubin C. Low-level, high-frequency mechanical signals enhance musculoskeletal development of young women with low BMD. J Bone Miner Res. 2006 Sep;21(9):1464-74.

34. Gusi N, Raimundo A, Leal A. Low-frequency vibratory exercise reduces the risk of bone fracture more than walking: a randomized controlled trial. BMC Musculoskeletal Disord. 2006 Nov 30;7:92.

35. Hagbarth K, Kunesch E. Gamma loop contributing to maximal voluntary contractions in man.
The journal of physiology 1986; 380(1): 575-591.

36. Jackson KJ, Merriman HL, Vanderburgh PM, Brahler CJ. Acute effects of whole-body vibration on lower extremity muscle performance in persons with multiple sclerosis. J Neurol Phys Ther. 2008 Dec;32(4):171-6.

37. Jacobs PL, Burns P. Acute enhancement of lower-extremity dynamic strength and flexibility with whole-body vibration. J Strength Cond Res. 2009 Jan;23(1):51-7.

38. Kasai T, Yahgi S, Shimura K. Effect of vibration-induced postural illusion on anticipatory postural adjustment of voluntary arm movement in standing humans. Gait posture 2002; 15(1): 94-100.

39. Kawanabe K, Kawashima A, Sashimoto I, Takeda T, Sato Y, Iwamoto J. Effect of whole-body vibration exercise and muscle strengthening, balance, and walking exercises on walking ability in the elderly. Keio J Med. 2007 Mar;56(1):28-33.

40. Kerschan-Schindl K, Grampp S, Resch H, Henk C, Preisinger E, Fialka-Moser V, Imhof H. Whole-body vibration exercise leads to alterations in muscle blood volume. Clinical physiology 2001; 21(3): 377-382.

41. Kinser AM, Ramsey MW, O'Bryant HS, Ayres CA, Sands WA, Stone MH. Vibration and stretching effects on flexibility and explosive strength in young gymnasts. Med Sci Sports Exerc. 2008 Jan;40(1):133-40.

42. Lamont HS, Cramer JT, Bemben DA, Shehab RL, Anderson MA, Bemben MG. Effects of 6 weeks of periodized squat training with or without whole-body vibration on short-term adaptations in jump performance within recreationally resistance trained men. J Strength Cond Res. 2008 Nov;22(6):1882-93.

43. Luo J, Clarke M, McNamara B, Moran K. Influence of resistance load on neuromuscular response to vibration training. J Strength Cond Res. 2009 Mar;23(2):420-6.

44. Luo J, McNamara B, Moran K. Effect of vibration training on neuromuscular output with ballistic knee extensions. J Sports Sci. 2008 Oct;26(12):1365-73.

45. Luo J, McNamara B, Moran K. The use of vibration training to enhance muscle strength and power. Sports med 2005; 35(1): 23-40.

46. Lythgo N, Eser P, de Groot P, Galea M. Whole-body vibration dosage alters leg blood flow. Clin Physiol Funct Imaging. 2009; Jan;29(1):53-9.

47. Maddalozzo GF, Iwaniec UT, Turner RT, Rosen CJ, Widrick JJ. Whole-body vibration slows the acquisition of fat in mature female rats. Int J Obes (Lond). 2008 Sep;32(9):1348-54. Epub 2008 Jul 29.

48. Mahieu NN, Witvrouw E, Van de Voorde D, Michilsens D, Arbyn V, Van den Broecke W. Improving strength and postural control in young skiers: whole-body vibration versus equivalent resistance training. J Athl Train. 2006 Jul-Sep;41(3):286-93.

49. Mileva KN, Bowtell JL, Kossev AR. Effects of low-frequency whole-body vibration on motor-evoked potentials in healthy men. Exp Physiol. 2009 Jan;94(1):103-16. Epub 2008 Jul 25.

50. Mischi M, Cardinale M. The effects of a 28-Hz vibration on arm muscle activity during isometric exercise. Med Sci Sports Exerc. 2009 Mar;41(3):645-53.

51. Moran K, McNamara B, Luo J. Effect of vibration training in maximal effort (70% 1RM) dynamic bicep curls. Med Sci Sports Exerc. 2007 Mar;39(3):526-33.

52. Otsuki T, Takanami Y, Aoi W, Kawai Y, Ichikawa H, Yoshikawa T. Arterial stiffness acutely decreases after whole-body vibration in humans. Acta Physiol (Oxf). 2008 Nov;194(3):189-94. Epub 2008 Apr 30.

53. Oullier O, Kavounoudias A, Duclos C, Albert F, Roll JP, Roll R. Countering postural posteffects following prolonged exposure to whole-body vibration: a sensorimotor treatment. Eur J Appl Physiol. 2009 Jan;105(2):235-45. Epub 2008 Oct 31.

54. Rees SS, Murphy AJ, Watsford ML. Effects of whole body vibration on postural steadiness in an older population. J Sci Med Sport. 2008 Jun 10. [Epub ahead of print]

55. Rees SS, Murphy AJ, Watsford ML. Effects of whole-body vibration exercise on lower-extremity muscle strength and power in an older population: a randomized clinical trial. Phys Ther. 2008 Apr;88(4):462-70. Epub 2008 Jan 24.

56. Rehn B, Lidstrom J, Skoglund J, Lindstrom B. Effects on leg muscular performance from whole-body vibration exercise: a systematic review. Scand J Med Sci Sports. 2007 Feb;17(1):2-11. Epub 2006 Aug 10. Review.

57. Rietschel E, van Koningsbruggen S, Fricke O, Semler O, Schoenau E. Whole body vibration: a new therapeutic approach to improve muscle function in cystic fibrosis? Int J Rehabil Res. 2008 Sep;31(3):253-6.

58. Rittweger J, Just K, Kautzsch K, Reeg P, Felsenberg D. Treatment of chronic lower back pain with lumbar extension and whole-body vibration exercise. Spine 2002; 27(17): 1829-1834.

59. Roelants M, Verschueren SM, Delecluse C, Levin O, Stijnen V. Whole-body-vibration-induced increase in leg muscle activity during different squat exercises. J Strength Cond Res. 2006 Feb;20(1):124-9.

60. Roth J, Wust M, Rawer R, Schnabel D, Armbrecht G, Beller G, Rembitzki I, Wahn U, Felsenberg D, Staab D. Whole body vibration in cystic fibrosis - a pilot study. J Musculoskelet Neuronal Interact. 2008; Apr-Jun;8(2):179-87.

61. Rubin C, Pope M, Fritton J, Transmissibility of 15-hertz to 35-hertz vibrations to the human hip and lumbar spine: determining the physiologic feasibility of delivering low-level anabolic mechanical stimuli to skeletal regions at greatest risk of fracture because of osteoporosis. Spine 2003; 28(23): 2621-2627.

62. Trans T, Aaboe J, Henriksen M, Christensen R, Bliddal H, Lund H. Effect of whole body vibration exercise on muscle strength and proprioception in females with knee osteoarthritis. Knee. 2009 Jan 13. [Epub ahead of print]

63. van Nes IJ, Latour H, Schils F, Meijer R, van Kuijk A, Geurts AC. Long-term effects of 6-week whole-body vibration on balance recovery and activities of daily living in the postacute phase of stroke: a randomized, controlled trial. Stroke. 2006 Sep;37(9):2331- 5. Epub 2006 Aug 10.

64. Verschueren S, Roelants M, Delecluse C, Swinnen S, Vanderschueren D, Boonen S. Effect of 6-month whole body vibration training on hip density, muscle strength, and postural control in postmenopausal women: a randomized controlled pilot study. Journal of bone and mineral research 2004; 19(3): 352-359.

65. Wilcock IM, Whatman C, Harris N, Keogh JW. Vibration training: could it enhance the strength, power, or speed of athletes. J Strength Cond Res. 2009 Mar;23(2):593-603.

66. Fitness Treatment System. The newest concept fitness-treatment complex system. The Newest Concept JET-VIBE. Jet-Vibe manual.

www.ingramcontent.com/pod-product-compliance
Lightning Source LLC
Chambersburg PA
CBHW042346030426
42335CB00031B/3480